POWER OF ATTORNEY AND GUARDIANSHIP

POWER OF ATTORNEY AND GUARDIANSHIP

A GUIDE FOR FAMILIES AND HEALTHCARE PERSONNEL

KATIE DEWERDT, MS, CHES-R, LNHA

PHOTOGRAPHY BY
PIXABY.COM

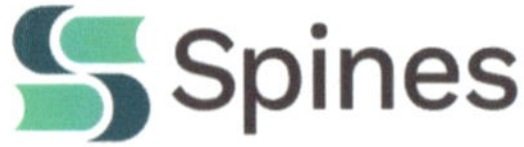

CONTENTS

PRELUDE AND ABOUT THE AUTHOR:

My name is Katie DeWerdt. I have a Master's in Science with a concentration in Cardiac Rehabilitation, Bachelor's in Science with a concentration in Community Health Education, Associate in Arts and a Certificate Degree in Website Development. I am also a Certified Health Education Specialist and Licensed Nursing Home Administrator. I have two published books. I have been working as an Administrator of Skilled nursing facilities since 2008. During this time, it is evident that many families struggle with the knowledge they need during difficult times when loved ones become incapacitated to make decisions on their own.

I am writing this guide to ensure that loved ones can take action and make informed decisions during times when their elderly are unable to make their own decisions. This guide can be helpful for other parties as well. For example, if someone has an accident and is no longer able to make decisions either financially or health-related, this book is a great guide to help in those circumstances as well. Or perhaps you are planning for your own future. It is important to know how to put those in power of your health and estate when your own health fails. Appointing the correct person or people can be a relief to ensure all things will be handled the way you would like.

POWER OF ATTORNEY AND GUARDIANSHIP

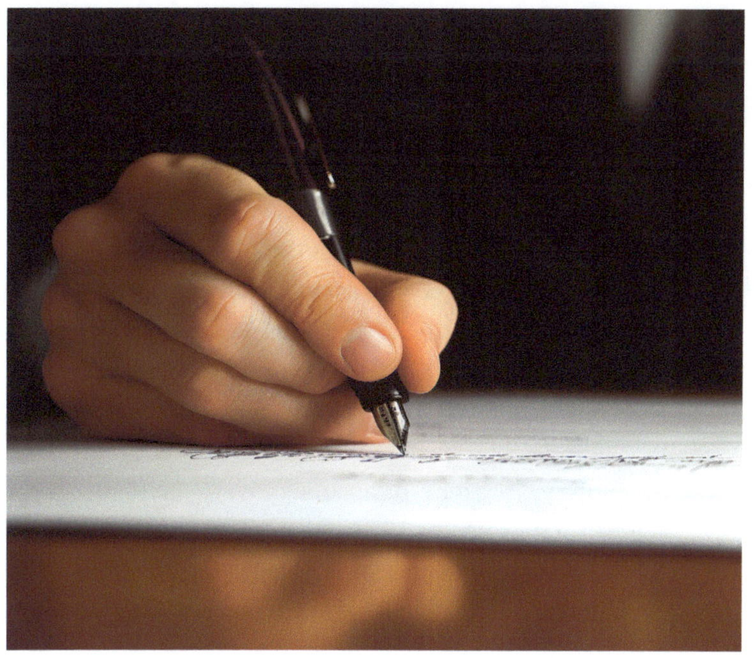

POWER OF ATTORNEY:

How many types of Power of Attorney are there?

There are several types of Power of Attorney (POA), each serving different purposes. The main types include:

1. **General Power of Attorney**: Gives broad powers to the agent to act on behalf of the principal in a variety of matters.
2. **Special or Limited Power of Attorney**: Allows the agent to act on behalf of the principal in specific situations or for particular tasks, such as selling a property.
3. **Durable Power of Attorney**: Remains in effect even if the principal becomes incapacitated. This type can be general or limited.
4. **Springing Power of Attorney**: Becomes effective only when a specified event occurs, typically when the principal becomes incapacitated.
5. **Healthcare Power of Attorney**: Specifically grants the agent authority to make healthcare decisions on behalf of the principal if they are incapacitated.
6. **Financial Power of Attorney**: Authorizes the agent to handle financial matters, such as managing bank accounts, paying bills, or handling investments.
7. **Revocation of Power of Attorney**: While not a type of POA itself, it's important to note that a principal can revoke any previously granted Power of Attorney at any time, provided they are still competent.

Each type serves different needs and legal requirements, and it's important to choose the one that aligns with your personal circumstances.

Throughout the next parts of this guide, you will get step-by-step information on how to attain power of attorney and how each type of power of attorney works.

GENERAL POWER OF ATTORNEY

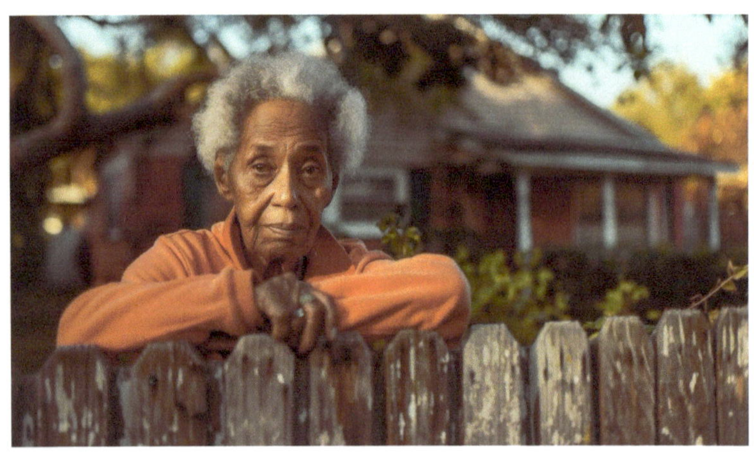

What is General Power of Attorney?

A General Power of Attorney (POA) is a legal document that grants an agent (also known as an attorney-in-fact) broad authority to act on behalf of the principal (the person granting the power). This document allows the agent to make a wide range of decisions and take various actions concerning the principal's financial, legal, and business affairs.

Key features of a General Power of Attorney include:

1. **Broad Authority:** The agent typically has the authority to handle nearly all financial and legal matters, which may include managing bank accounts, paying bills, filing taxes, purchasing or selling property, and making investment decisions.
2. **Legal Status:** The General POA is a legally binding document and usually must be signed in accordance with state laws, which may include witnessing and notarization requirements.
3. **Durability:** A General Power of Attorney can be durable or non-durable. If it is durable, it remains effective even if the principal becomes incapacitated. If it is non-durable, it ceases to be effective if the principal becomes incapacitated.
4. **Termination:** The General Power of Attorney can be revoked by the principal at any time, provided they are still competent. It may also terminate upon the death of the principal.
5. **Use Cases:** It is often used in situations where the principal is unable to manage their affairs due to travel, illness, or other personal circumstances.

It's crucial for both the principal and the agent to understand the responsibilities that come with a General Power of Attorney, as the agent will be trusted to make decisions in the best interest of the principal.

If the principal is intact, is General Power of Attorney in effect?

Yes, if the principal is intact (i.e., fully competent and able to make decisions). In that case, a General Power of Attorney is typically in effect, provided that it has been properly executed (signed and notarized, if required) and has not been revoked.

The General Power of Attorney allows the agent to act on the principal's behalf in various matters as specified in the document. However, the principal retains the ability to manage their own affairs and can revoke or modify the POA at any time while they are still competent. In essence, the General Power of Attorney complements the principal's ability to act but does not replace it unless the principal chooses to delegate specific responsibilities to the agent.

WHAT FORMS NEEDS TO BE SIGNED FOR GENERAL POWER OF ATTORNEY TO TAKE PLACE?

To create a General Power of Attorney (POA), certain forms and steps need to be followed. Here's an overview of the typical requirements:

1. **General Power of Attorney Document:** You will need a legal document that outlines the powers granted to the agent. This document should include:
   - The names of the principal and the agent.
   - A statement granting the agent authority to act on behalf of the principal.
   - A list of specific powers granted to the agent (e.g., financial decisions, property management).
   - Any limitations or conditions applicable to the agent's authority.
   - The effective date of the POA.
2. **Signatures:** The principal must sign the General Power of Attorney document. Depending on state laws, the agent may also need to sign to accept the designation.

3. **Witnesses:** Many states require that the General POA be signed in the presence of one or more witnesses. The number of required witnesses can vary by state.

4. **Notarization:** Most states require the General Power of Attorney to be notarized to be considered valid. This means that a notary public must witness the signing of the document and affix their seal to it.

5. **State-Specific Requirements:** It's important to check the specific requirements in your state, as laws regarding POAs can vary significantly. Some states may have their own forms or additional requirements that must be met.

6. **Copy Distribution:** After executing the POA, it is recommended that copies be provided to the agent, financial institutions, healthcare providers, and any other relevant parties who may need access to the document.

It's advisable to consult with an attorney or legal professional to ensure that the General Power of Attorney document meets all legal requirements and effectively reflects the principal's intentions.

Please note that skilled nursing facility personnel can help with healthcare power of attorney paperwork as long as the resident is not demented. Usually, social services can help with this; however, skilled nursing facilities cannot be involved in General Power of Attorney documents because it includes financial responsibilities.

Are General Power of Attorney Forms legal even if a lawyer did not generate them?

Yes, a General Power of Attorney (POA) form can still be considered legal even if it was not generated by a lawyer, as long as the document meets the legal requirements set forth by the state where it is executed. However, there are several important considerations:

1. **State Laws:** Each state has specific laws governing the creation and execution of a Power of Attorney. The form must comply with these laws, including proper wording, format, and required signatures.

2. **Execution Requirements:** The document usually needs to be signed by the principal and may require one or more witnesses and notarization, depending on state laws. Failure to adhere to these requirements can result in the document being deemed invalid.

3. **Clarity and Specificity:** It's crucial that the form clearly specifies the authority granted to the agent and any limitations. Vague or ambiguous language can lead to confusion or disputes in the future.

4. **Risks of DIY Forms:** While using a template or DIY form can save costs, there is a risk of accidentally including incorrect language, failing to include necessary provisions, or not complying with state requirements. This could lead to the POA being challenged or invalidated.

5. **Best Practice:** It's generally advisable to consult with a legal professional when creating important legal documents like a Power of Attorney. An attorney can ensure that the document is properly drafted and meets all legal requirements for validity, helping to avoid potential issues down the line.

In summary, while a General Power of Attorney form created without a lawyer can be legal, it is essential to ensure that it complies with the relevant state laws and requirements.

WHAT IS SPECIAL OR LIMITED POWER OF ATTORNEY?

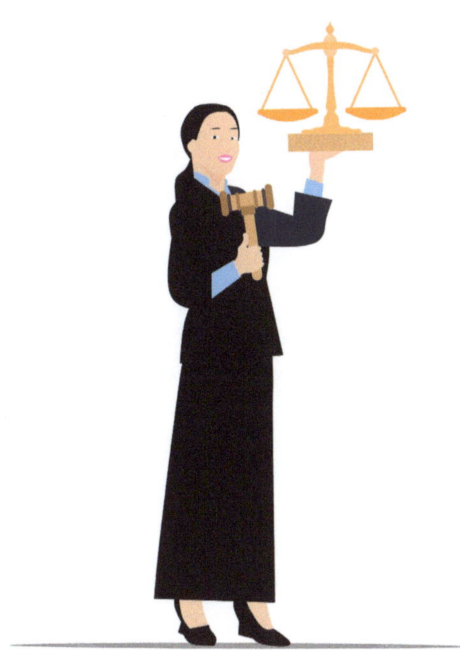

A Special Power of Attorney, also known as a Limited Power of Attorney, is a legal document that grants an agent (attorney-in-fact) authority to act on behalf of the principal (the person granting the power) only in specific situations or for designated tasks. This type of POA is more restricted compared to a General Power of Attorney, which provides broader authority.

Key Features of Special or Limited Power of Attorney:

1. **Specific Authority:** The agent's powers are limited to the specific actions or decisions explicitly outlined in the document. For example, the agent may be authorized to sell a particular property, handle a specific financial transaction, or make decisions regarding a particular legal matter.
2. **Duration:** The Special Power of Attorney can be set to be effective for a limited time or until a specific event occurs. For example, it could be used for a particular transaction or only during the principal's absence.
3. **Execution Requirements:** Like other types of Power of Attorney, a Special Power of Attorney must be properly executed according to state laws, which may include signatures from the principal, witnesses, and notarization.
4. **Revocation:** The principal can revoke a Special Power of Attorney at any time, provided they are still competent to do so. This revocation should be documented formally, and copies should be distributed to relevant parties.
5. **Common Use Cases:** Special Power of Attorney is commonly used in situations such as:

- Selling or managing a specific property or asset.
- Completing a business transaction when the principal cannot be present.
- Handling financial matters or preferences related to a specific event, such as a real estate closing.
- Making healthcare decisions in limited circumstances, though this is more commonly handled by a Healthcare Power of Attorney.

In summary, Special or Limited Power of Attorney is a versatile legal tool that allows a principal to delegate authority for specific tasks or decisions while maintaining control over other matters. It is essential to clearly outline the scope of the agent's authority to avoid confusion or misuse.

WHAT FORMS ARE NEEDED FOR SPECIAL OR LIMITED POWER OF ATTORNEY?

Creating a Special or Limited Power of Attorney (POA) typically requires a specific form that outlines the powers granted to the agent (attorney-in-fact). The forms and requirements can vary by state, but generally, the following components are needed:

1. Special Power of Attorney Document:

- A legal document that clearly states:
    - The names of the principal and the agent.
    - The specific powers being granted to the agent (e.g., selling a particular property, managing financial accounts for a specified transaction).
    - The effective date of the POA and any expiration date or conditions under which it becomes ineffective.
    - Any limitations on the agent's authority.

2. Signatures:

- The principal must sign the Special Power of Attorney document. The agent typically does not need to sign the document to make it valid, but it is often included to acknowledge acceptance of the role.

3. Witnesses:

- Many states require that the POA be signed in the presence of one or more witnesses. The number of required witnesses may vary by state.

4. Notarization:

- Most states require the Special Power of Attorney to be notarized. A notary public must witness the signing of the document and provide their seal.

5. State-Specific Requirements:

- It's crucial to check the specific laws in the state where the POA will be executed, as some states may have unique forms, additional requirements, or statutory language that must be included.

6. Distribution of Copies:

- After the POA is executed, it is advisable to provide copies to the agent and any institutions or parties that may need to recognize the authority, such as banks, real estate companies, or healthcare providers.

Conclusion:

While it is possible to find templates for a Special or Limited Power of Attorney online, it is highly recommended to consult with a legal professional to ensure that the document meets all legal requirements and properly reflects the principal's intentions. This helps prevent misunderstandings and complications later on.

WHAT IS A DURABLE POWER OF ATTORNEY?

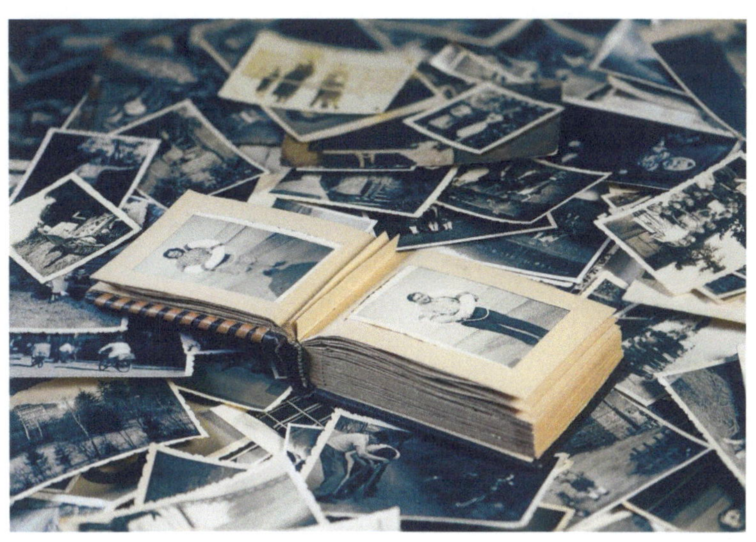

A Durable Power of Attorney (POA) is a specific type of Power of Attorney that remains in effect even if the principal (the person granting the power) becomes incapacitated or unable to make decisions for themselves. This contrasts with a non-durable Power of Attorney, which becomes invalid upon the principal's incapacitation.

Key Features of Durable Power of Attorney:

1. **Continuation of Authority:** A Durable Power of Attorney allows the agent (attorney-in-fact) to continue acting on behalf of the principal even in the event of the principal's incapacity. This can be crucial for managing financial and legal matters without interruption.
2. **Scope of Authority:** The durable POA can be general (granting broad powers) or limited (focusing on specific tasks or situations). The principal must clearly define the extent of the agent's authority in the document.
3. **Execution Requirements:** Like other forms of POA, a Durable Power of Attorney must be properly executed according to state laws, which generally require:
    - The principal's signature.
    - Possible witnesses (depending on state requirements).
    - Notarization (in most states).
4. **Revocation:** The principal can revoke a Durable Power of Attorney at any time, as long as they are still competent. Once revoked, the agent no longer has the authority to act on behalf of the principal.

5. **Common Use Cases:** Durable Powers of Attorney are commonly utilized for:
    - Planning for potential future incapacitation (e.g., due to illness, injury, or aging).
    - Managing finances, property, and medical decisions in the event the principal can no longer do so themselves.

6. **Healthcare Durable Power of Attorney:** It's important to note that there's often a specific type of durable POA designated for healthcare decisions, sometimes called a Healthcare Power of Attorney or Durable Power of Attorney for Health Care. This form allows the agent to make medical decisions on behalf of the principal if they are unable to do so.

Importance of Durable Power of Attorney:

Having a Durable Power of Attorney in place can provide peace of mind, knowing that someone trusted can manage affairs and make decisions in case the principal can no longer do so. It's essential to select an agent who is responsible and reliable, as they will have significant authority over the principal's financial and legal matters.

Consulting with a legal professional is advisable to ensure that the Durable Power of Attorney is properly drafted and meets all legal requirements specific to your state.

In healthcare settings, durable power of attorney is helpful. There are decisions that healthcare clinicians can not make for individuals. For example, if a person is unable to take nutrients by mouth for any reason and is unable to make their own decisions, healthcare personnel cannot make this decision. A power

of attorney is needed. For psychotropic medications, someone must give consent. When a person is unable to make their own decisions, durable power of attorney is helpful. When deciding on a power of attorney for your own needs, ensure that the person taking responsibility knows what you want. For example, do you want to be placed on a ventilator if one is necessary? These questions are important to discuss with your power of attorney. Healthcare power of attorney will be discussed.

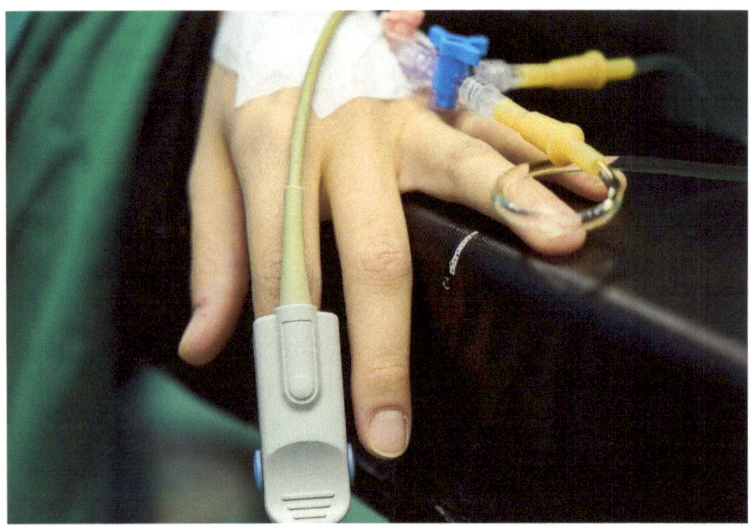

WHAT FORMS ARE NEEDED FOR DURABLE POWER OF ATTORNEY?

Creating a Durable Power of Attorney (POA) typically requires specific forms and adherence to certain procedures. The requirements can vary by state, but generally, the following components are needed:

1. Durable Power of Attorney Document:

- A legal document that explicitly states:
  - The names of the principal (the person granting the power) and the agent (attorney-in-fact).
  - A clear declaration that the POA is durable, indicating it will remain effective even if the principal becomes incapacitated.
  - The specific powers granted to the agent—these might be broad (financial and legal decisions) or limited (specific tasks).
  - Any limitations on the authority of the agent, if applicable.
  - The effective date of the POA.

2. Signatures:

- The principal must sign the Durable Power of Attorney form. The agent usually does not need to sign the document but may do so to acknowledge acceptance of the role.

3. Witnesses:

- Many states require that the Durable Power of Attorney be signed in the presence of one or more witnesses. The number of witnesses varies by state, so check your local requirements.

4. Notarization:

- Most states require the Durable Power of Attorney to be notarized. A notary public must witness the signing of the document and provide their seal to validate it.

5. State-Specific Requirements:

- It's important to check the specific laws of your state, as some states may have their own forms or additional requirements that must be met for the Durable Power of Attorney to be valid.

6. Distribution of Copies:

- After the document is executed, it's a good idea to provide copies to:
  - The agent named in the POA.

  o Financial institutions, healthcare providers, and
    any relevant parties that may need to recognize
    the authority granted.

Conclusion:

While templates for Durable Power of Attorney forms can often be found online, it is highly recommended to consult with a legal professional to ensure that the form meets all legal requirements and accurately reflects the principal's intentions. This proactive step can help prevent potential issues or disputes in the future.

HOW MUCH DOES IT COST TO HAVE DURABLE POWER OF ATTORNEY PAPERWORK DRAWN UP?

The cost of having Durable Power of Attorney (POA) paperwork drawn up can vary widely based on several factors, including:

1. **Location:** Legal fees can differ significantly by region or state. Urban areas may have higher legal costs than rural areas.
2. **Attorney Fees:** If you hire an attorney to draft the Durable Power of Attorney, costs typically range from $100 to $500 or more, depending on the attorney's experience, reputation, and the complexity of your needs.
3. **Service Rates:** Some legal services or online platforms may offer pre-made templates or document preparation services for a lower fee, generally ranging from $20 to $150. However, using a template does not provide personalized legal advice.
4. **Complexity of the Document:** If your situation requires more customized provisions or complex legal language, the cost may increase.

5. **Notarization and Witness Fees:** Notarization may incur an additional fee, which can range from $5 to $20 per signature, and if witnesses are needed, they may charge a nominal fee as well.

Estimated Costs Summary:

- Attorney Fees: $100 to $500+
- Online Templates/Services: $20 to $150
- Notary Fees: $5 to $20 per signature

Conclusion:

Overall, having a Durable Power of Attorney drafted by a qualified attorney tends to provide greater assurance that the document will be properly executed and legally valid, especially for more complex situations. It's advisable to shop around, get quotes, and potentially consult multiple legal professionals to find the best option that meets your needs and budget. If your situation is straightforward, you might also consider using an online service to create a POA at a lower cost.

Families need to discuss these arrangements prior to incapacitation. During highly emotional times, these decisions can be very difficult to manage. Having these discussions ahead of time and putting the proper person in authority is an important step to ensure that your wishes are being completed during incapacitation. Having a durable power of attorney can allow your wishes to be carried out.

Healthcare personnel at skilled nursing facilities cannot create durable power of attorney forms for families because it includes financial decisions as well as healthcare decisions.

WHAT IS SPRINGING POWER OF ATTORNEY?

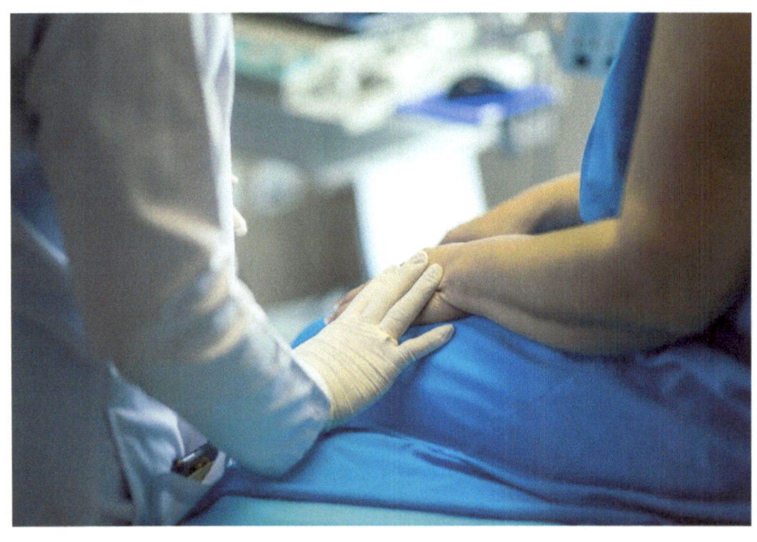

A Springing Power of Attorney is a specific type of Power of Attorney (POA) that becomes effective only upon the occurrence of a specified event, typically the incapacitation of the principal (the person who grants the authority). This means that the agent (attorney-in-fact) does not have authority to act on behalf of the principal until that specified condition is met.

Key Features of Springing Power of Attorney:

1. **Conditional Effectiveness:** The authority granted to the agent is activated only when the principal becomes incapacitated or unable to manage their affairs, as defined in the document. This can provide peace of mind to the principal, as they maintain control until they need assistance.
2. **Specific Trigger Event:** The document clearly outlines the event or condition that triggers the agent's authority. It's important for the trigger to be well-defined to prevent ambiguity and potential disputes.
3. **Durability:** A Springing POA can be drafted to be a durable power of attorney, meaning it will remain in effect even if the principal becomes incapacitated after it is activated.
4. **Execution Requirements:** Like other types of POAs, a Springing Power of Attorney must comply with state laws, which typically require signatures, potential witnesses, and notarization to be valid.
5. **Common Use Cases:** Springing Powers of Attorney are often used in estate planning, where individuals want to retain control over their personal and financial matters until it is truly necessary to delegate authority to another person.

6. **Assessment of Incapacity:** The POA document should ideally outline how incapacity will be determined (e.g., a written opinion from a physician) to provide clarity and avoid disputes regarding the agent's authority.

Advantages of Springing Power of Attorney:

- **Control:** The principal retains full control and autonomy over their decisions until a predetermined event occurs.
- **Avoids Immediate Authority:** The agent does not have powers until the specified conditions are met, which can be reassuring for the principal.

Disadvantages of Springing Power of Attorney:

- **Potential Delays:** Activation may require assessments or documentation that could delay the agent's ability to act when quick decisions are necessary.
- **Complexity:** Setting up a Springing POA can be more complex than a general or durable POA, particularly in defining conditions and ensuring compliance with legal requirements.

Conclusion:

A Springing Power of Attorney can be a valuable estate planning tool for individuals looking to maintain control of their affairs while preparing for potential future incapacity. It's advisable to consult with an attorney or legal professional to ensure that the document is properly drafted and meets all legal requirements.

WHAT FORMS ARE NEEDED FOR SPRINGING POWER OF ATTORNEY?

Creating a Springing Power of Attorney (POA) typically requires specific forms and adherence to certain legal requirements. The requirements can vary by state, but generally, the following components are needed:

1. Springing Power of Attorney Document:

- **A legal document that clearly states:**
  - The names of the principal (the person granting the power) and the agent (attorney-in-fact).
  - A clear declaration that this is a Springing Power of Attorney, along with the specific event or condition that will trigger the agent's authority (usually the incapacitation of the principal).
  - The specific powers being granted to the agent—these might be broad (general financial and legal decisions) or limited (specific tasks).
  - Any limitations on the agent's authority, if applicable.

- Instructions on how incapacity will be determined (e.g., by a physician's assessment).

2. Signatures:

- The principal must sign the Springing Power of Attorney form. Depending on state requirements, the agent may also sign the document to acknowledge acceptance of the role.

3. Witnesses:

- Many states require that the Springing Power of Attorney be signed in the presence of one or more witnesses. The number of required witnesses can vary, so it's essential to check your local laws.

4. Notarization:

- Most states require the Springing Power of Attorney to be notarized. A notary public must witness the signing of the document and provide their seal, validating the document.

5. State-Specific Requirements:

- It's critical to review the specific laws in your state, as variations exist regarding the required language, forms, and execution procedures for Power of Attorney documents.

6. Distribution of Copies:

- After the document is executed, it's a good idea to distribute copies to:
  - The agent named in the POA.
  - Any institutions (banks, healthcare providers, etc.) that may need to recognize the authority granted.
  - Family members who may need to be aware of the arrangement.

Conclusion:

While there may be templates for a Springing Power of Attorney available online, it's highly advisable to consult with a legal professional to ensure that the document is properly drafted to meet legal requirements and accurately reflects the principal's intentions. This can help prevent misunderstandings or disputes in the future.

WHAT IS HEALTHCARE POWER OF ATTORNEY?

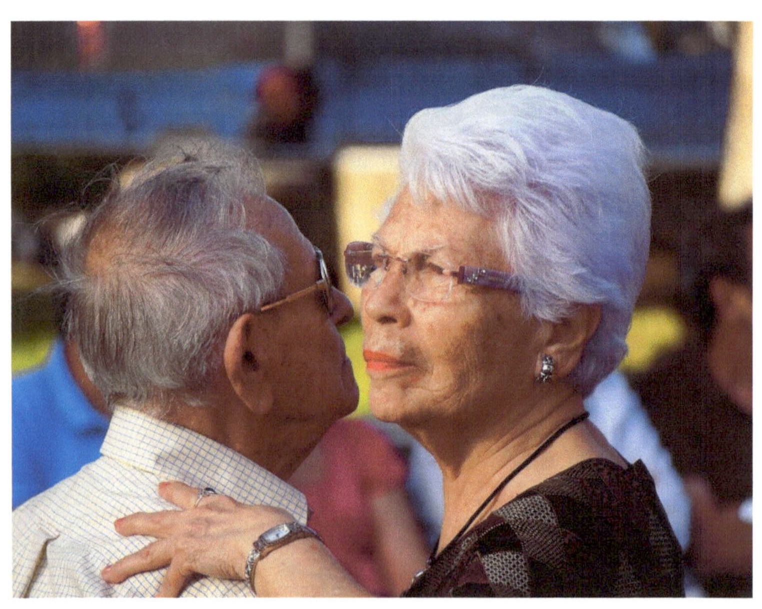

A Healthcare Power of Attorney (Healthcare POA) is a legal document that allows an individual (the principal) to designate another person (the agent or attorney-in-fact) to make healthcare decisions on their behalf in the event that they become unable to communicate their wishes or make decisions due to illness, injury, or incapacitation.

Key Features of Healthcare Power of Attorney:

1. **Authority for Healthcare Decisions:** The primary function of a Healthcare POA is to grant the agent the authority to make medical decisions for the principal, including choices about treatments, procedures, and end-of-life care.
2. **Specific Instructions:** The document may include specific instructions regarding the principal's healthcare preferences. This can involve the types of medical treatments they would want or refuse, making their wishes clear to the agent.
3. **Activation of Authority:** Typically, the authority of the agent becomes effective when the principal is deemed incapacitated by a qualified medical professional. Some states may have different rules regarding how and when the authority is activated.
4. **Compliance with State Laws:** Healthcare POA documents must comply with the laws and requirements of the state in which they are executed, including any necessary language, signatures, and notarization or witness requirements.
5. **Revocation:** The principal can revoke a Healthcare Power of Attorney at any time while they are still competent. This can be done through a clear written statement or by executing a new POA.

6. **Common Use Cases:** A Healthcare POA is commonly used in situations such as:
   - Hospitals or medical facilities when a patient is unconscious or otherwise unable to voice their wishes.
   - Long-term care decisions, including nursing home placement or hospice care.
   - Emergency situations where immediate healthcare decisions are needed.

Importance of Healthcare Power of Attorney:

Having a Healthcare Power of Attorney is essential for ensuring that your healthcare preferences are honored, particularly in situations where you may not be able to communicate them yourself. It provides peace of mind that a trusted individual will be available to make critical health decisions based on your wishes.

Conclusion:

A Healthcare Power of Attorney is a vital component of effective healthcare planning. Consulting with a legal professional is advisable to accurately draft the document, ensuring compliance with state laws while reflecting the principal's values and preferences regarding healthcare decisions.

Although consulting a legal professional is advisable, there are situations where quick decisions need to be made for one's healthcare choices. Skilled Nursing Facilities and Hospitals should be able to guide families to fill out healthcare power of attorney under the condition that the person is of sound mind and does not have dementia. That is why the importance of deciding healthcare power of attorney should be determined before illnesses strike.

WHAT FORMS ARE NEEDED FOR HEALTHCARE POWER OF ATTORNEY?

Creating Power of Attorney (Healthcare POA) typically involves specific forms and adherence to legal requirements that can vary by state. Generally, the following components are needed:

1. Healthcare Power of Attorney Document:

- **A legal document that clearly states:**
  - The principal's name (the person granting the authority).
  - The agent's name (the individual designated to make healthcare decisions).
  - A clear declaration that the document serves as a Healthcare Power of Attorney.
  - The specific authorities granted to the agent may include making decisions regarding medical treatment, surgery, medication, and end-of-life care.
  - Any specific wishes or instructions regarding healthcare treatment, if desired.

2. Signatures:

- The principal must sign the Healthcare Power of Attorney document. In some cases, the agent may also sign to acknowledge their acceptance of the role, but this is not always required.

3. Witnesses:

- Many states require that the Healthcare Power of Attorney be signed in the presence of one or more witnesses. The number of required witnesses can vary by state, so it's important to verify the local requirements.

4. Notarization:

- While not required in all states, many jurisdictions do require that the Healthcare POA be notarized. A notary public will witness the signing of the document and affix their seal to verify its authenticity.

5. State-Specific Requirements:

- It is essential to check the specific laws in your state, as there may be unique forms, wording, or additional requirements that must be satisfied for a Healthcare Power of Attorney to be valid. Some states may have statutory forms that you can use.

6. Distribution of Copies:

- After the document is executed, it's advisable to
  provide copies to:
    - The agent designated in the document.
    - Family members who may need to be aware of
      the arrangement.
    - Medical providers, hospitals, and any relevant
      healthcare institutions to ensure they have access
      to the document when needed.

Conclusion:

Templates for healthcare power of attorney are available online. Also, most skilled nursing facilities and hospitals have forms families can fill out to ensure healthcare power of attorney is in place. If you are concerned about ensuring your specific wishes are carried out, then consult a legal representative.

In the coming paragraphs, we will discuss additional facts about healthcare power of attorney and state-specific guidelines for healthcare power of attorney. This is the type of power of attorney we will spend the most time on, as it is one of the most essential from my standpoint as an Administrator of a skilled nursing facility.

What Types Of Questions Should I Specify In Healthcare Power Of Attorney?

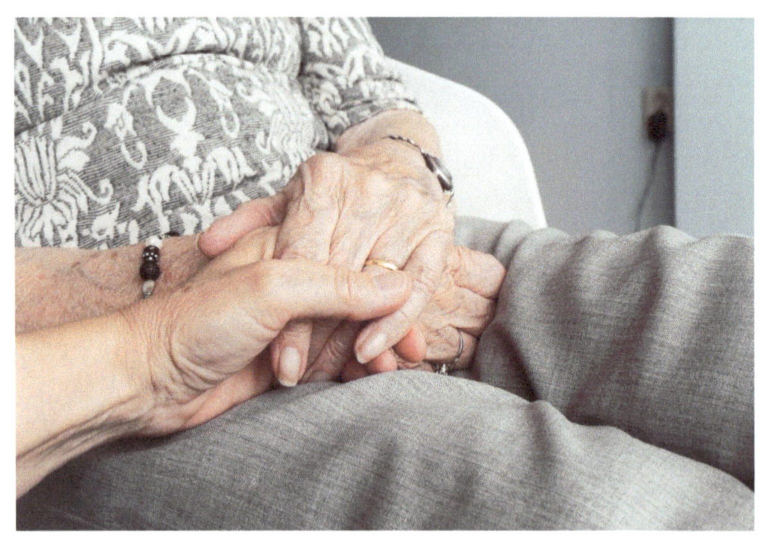

When drafting a Healthcare Power of Attorney (POA), it is important to consider various questions and scenarios to ensure that your wishes regarding medical treatment are clearly understood and can be effectively carried out by your appointed agent. Here are some key questions and areas to address:

1. General Healthcare Decisions:

- What types of medical treatments do you want to include or exclude?
- Are there specific procedures or interventions that you want to authorize or refuse (e.g., surgeries, hospitalizations)?

2. End-of-Life Decisions:

- What are your wishes regarding life-sustaining treatments (e.g., artificial nutrition and hydration, ventilators, resuscitation)?
- Under what circumstances would you want to discontinue life-sustaining measures?
- Do you want to receive palliative care or hospice care if you are terminally ill?

3. Specific Medical Conditions:

- Are there particular medical conditions under which you want your agent to make decisions (e.g., irreversible coma, advanced dementia)?
- How should your agent decide if you have a significant or terminal illness?

4. Organ Donation:

- Do you wish to donate your organs or tissues? If so, under what circumstances?
- Have you registered as an organ donor, and do you want that recorded in your Healthcare POA?

5. Mental Health Decisions:

- Do you have any specific instructions regarding mental health treatment or interventions (e.g., medications, hospitalization)?
- Would you want your agent to have authority over decisions related to mental health treatment?

6. Medication Preferences:

- Are there specific medications you would like to ensure you receive or avoid?
- What are your preferences regarding pain management and comfort care?

7. Consultation with Healthcare Providers:

- Do you authorize your agent to consult with healthcare providers and access your medical records?
- Are there specific individuals or types of healthcare professionals your agent should consult before making decisions?

8. Cultural or Religious Considerations:

- Are there any cultural or religious beliefs that should guide your healthcare decisions?
- Do you want your agent to consider spiritual or religious practices when making medical decisions on your behalf?

9. Communication with Family:

- Should your agent involve family members in healthcare decisions?
- How do you want your agent to handle communication about your condition with family members?

10. Scope of Authority:

- What specific powers do you want to grant to your agent? Are there any limitations you want to place on their authority?
- Do you want to specify how decisions should be made (e.g., based on known wishes and best interests)?

Conclusion:

It can be beneficial to have open and honest discussions with your appointed agent, family members, and healthcare providers about these questions before finalizing your Healthcare Power of Attorney. Documenting your preferences clearly in the POA will help guide your agent's decisions in alignment with your values and wishes during critical medical situations.

WHEN DOES A HEALTHCARE POWER OF ATTORNEY AGENT TAKE CHARGE OF DECISIONS?

A Healthcare Power of Attorney (POA) agent typically takes charge of making healthcare decisions on behalf of the principal (the person who granted the authority) under specific circumstances, primarily when the principal is deemed unable to make their own decisions. Here are the common scenarios outlining when the agent's authority begins:

1. Incapacity:

- The agent generally gains authority to make decisions when the principal is declared incapacitated. Incapacity often refers to situations where the principal is unable to comprehend or communicate their healthcare decisions effectively due to illness, injury, or a medical condition (such as being unconscious or having a severe cognitive impairment).

2. Medical Evaluation:

- Many states require a formal evaluation to determine incapacity before the agent can act. This evaluation is usually performed by one or more licensed healthcare professionals who will assess the principal's ability to make informed decisions regarding their health.

3. Specific Conditions Outlined in the POA:

- The Healthcare POA document may specify particular conditions under which the agent's authority becomes effective. For example, it may state that the agent can begin making decisions only after a specific medical diagnosis or condition is confirmed.

4. Agent's Authority:

- The authority granted to the agent can vary based on the language in the POA document. It is important for the principal to clearly outline the scope of authority and any limitations in the document, specifying whether the agent can override the principal's wishes if the principal becomes incapacitated.

5. Duration of Authority:

- The agent remains authorized to make healthcare decisions until one of the following occurs:
  - The principal regains the capacity to make decisions and revokes the authority.
  - The principal passes away (at which point the POA is no longer valid).

    o The POA is formally revoked or terminated by the principal, if competent.

Conclusion:

The activation of a Healthcare Power of Attorney is primarily centered around the principal's capacity to make informed healthcare decisions. Therefore, it is crucial for the principal to communicate their wishes clearly in the POA document and consider discussing these wishes with their chosen agent and family members. This helps ensure that the agent understands how to make decisions in alignment with the principal's values and preferences when the time comes.

In most states, a surrogate decision maker will be consulted in the event that there is no healthcare power of attorney set up. The surrogate decision maker is the closest relative or friend to the principal.

HOW DOES SURROGATE DECISION-MAKING WORK IN HEALTHCARE SETTINGS?

Surrogate decision-making in healthcare settings refers to the process by which a designated person (the surrogate) makes medical decisions on behalf of a patient who is unable to do so due to incapacity, such as unconsciousness, severe cognitive impairment, or other conditions affecting decision-making abilities. Here's how the process generally works:

1. Identification of the Surrogate:

- **Legal Designation**: If the patient has a Healthcare Power of Attorney, the appointed agent (attorney-in-fact) is typically the first authority for decision-making.
- **Surrogate Hierarchy**: In the absence of a designated agent, most states have laws that define a hierarchy of individuals who can serve as surrogates. This hierarchy often includes:
  - Spouse or domestic partner
  - Adult children
  - Parents

- Siblings
- Other close relatives or individuals familiar with the patient's values and wishes

2. Assessment of Incapacity:

- A healthcare professional (usually a physician) must determine that the patient is incapacitated and unable to make informed decisions about their medical care. This assessment often involves understanding the patient's medical condition, cognitive functioning, and ability to communicate.

3. Informed Decision-Making:

- The surrogate is responsible for making healthcare decisions based on the patient's wishes, values, and preferences. If the patient's wishes are unclear, the surrogate should act in the patient's best interest, considering the likely benefits and risks of proposed treatments.

4. Communication with Healthcare Providers:

- Surrogates typically work closely with healthcare providers to understand the patient's medical condition, treatment options, potential outcomes, and the implications of different choices. Effective communication is essential to ensure that surrogates make informed decisions.

5. Documentation:

- Decisions made by the surrogate may need to be documented in the patient's medical records, and healthcare providers may require confirmation of the surrogate's authority to act on the patient's behalf (e.g., a copy of the Healthcare POA or proof of surrogate status).

6. Legal Considerations:

- Surrogates are generally expected to follow state laws and hospital policies regarding decision-making authority. They should also be aware of any advance directives or written statements the patient may have expressed prior to incapacity.

7. Disagreements and Conflicts:

- In some cases, there may be disagreements among family members or between the healthcare team and the surrogate regarding treatment decisions. In such situations, healthcare providers may seek mediation or legal intervention to resolve disputes and ensure that the best interests of the patient are upheld.

8. End-of-Life Decisions:

- Surrogates may also be involved in making decisions about end-of-life care, including the use of life-sustaining treatments, palliative care, and hospice options. Being aware of the patient's values and wishes becomes critical in these sensitive situations.

Conclusion:

Surrogate decision-making is a vital component of healthcare for patients who cannot express their wishes. Having clear advance directives, such as a Healthcare Power of Attorney, can help clarify the patient's preferences and reduce potential conflicts or uncertainties regarding medical care. It is crucial for surrogates to communicate openly with healthcare providers and other family members and to base their decisions on the patient's values and previously stated wishes.

Surrogate decision-makers do have the authority to make sure no adverse decisions are being made for their loved ones. There was a time when my cousin was in the hospital, and the hospital was making poor choices for my cousin. I spoke to my aunt to empower her to utilize her authority as the surrogate decision-maker. If there is no healthcare power of attorney set up, the surrogate decision-maker has the power to ensure that the correct decisions are made for loved ones.

WHAT DECISIONS CANNOT BE MADE BY HEALTHCARE PERSONNEL?

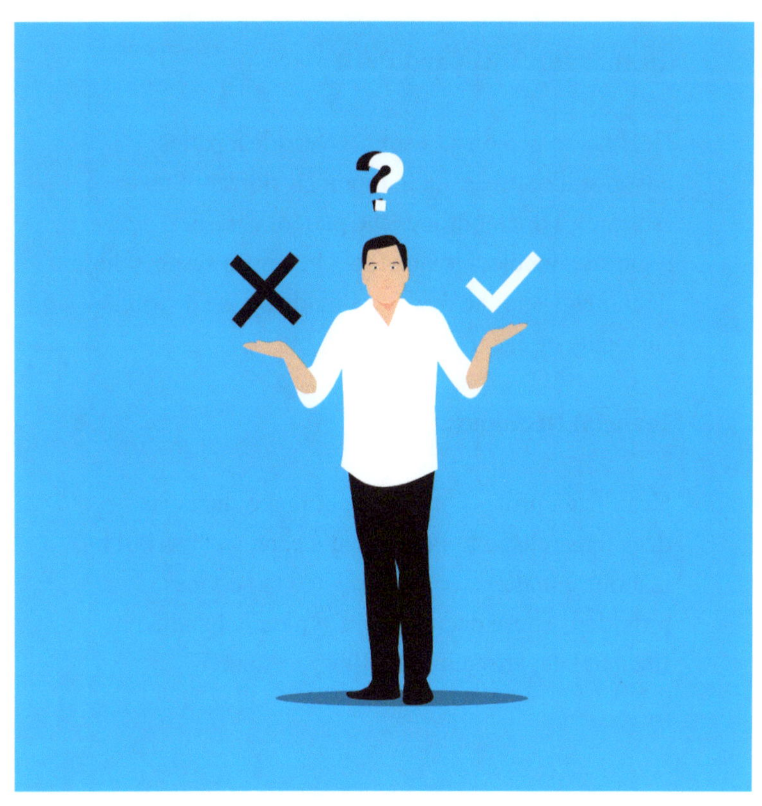

In healthcare settings, there are specific decisions that healthcare personnel (like doctors, nurses, and other medical staff) may not have the authority to make, either due to legal, ethical, or policy restrictions. Here are some key areas where healthcare personnel typically cannot make decisions:

1. Legal Competency Decisions:

- Healthcare professionals cannot determine the legal competency of a patient. This determination is usually made by a qualified legal or medical professional, often in conjunction with specific guidelines or legal standards.

2. Advance Directives and Preferences:

- Healthcare personnel cannot override a patient's advance directives, including a Healthcare Power of Attorney, which outlines the patient's wishes regarding medical treatment. They must respect these documents and the decisions made by the appointed surrogate or agent.

3. Financial Decisions:

- Healthcare professionals do not make financial decisions related to the patient's care, such as billing, insurance matters, or costs related to services provided. These decisions are typically handled by financial departments or billing personnel.

4. Treatment Against Medical Advice:

- While healthcare personnel can advise and recommend treatments, they cannot force treatments upon a patient who is clearly competent and chooses to refuse care or treatment (unless there are legal directives in place, such as court orders).

5. End-of-Life Decisions:

- While healthcare providers can discuss options regarding end-of-life care and offer guidance, they are generally not authorized to make unilateral decisions about whether to initiate, continue, or withdraw life-sustaining treatments. Such decisions must align with the patient's wishes, as expressed in advance directives, or should be made by the designated surrogate or legal representative.

6. Experimental Treatments:

- Healthcare providers cannot administer experimental treatments without informed consent from the patient or their surrogate. Patients must be fully informed about risks, benefits, and alternatives before agreeing to participate in experimental therapies.

7. Consent for Minors and Incompetent Persons:

- Healthcare personnel cannot make decisions regarding medical treatment for minors or those deemed incompetent without appropriate consent from a parent or legal guardian or from a designated surrogate decision-maker.

8. Transfer or Discharge Decisions:

- Decisions regarding transferring a patient to another facility or discharging them from a hospital may require institutional policies, physician orders, and appropriate patient consent. Healthcare personnel cannot unilaterally make these decisions without considering legal and ethical guidelines.

9. Treatment That Conflicts with Ethics or Policy:

- Healthcare personnel may not pursue treatments that conflict with hospital policies or ethical guidelines, such as requests for procedures that are outside the standard of care or deemed unnecessary.

Conclusion:

Healthcare personnel play a critical role in providing care and recommendations, but they must operate within the limits of legal, ethical, and institutional guidelines. Respecting patient autonomy, advance directives, and the authority of designated surrogates is crucial in ensuring ethical and lawful healthcare decisions. Open communication about the patient's wishes and legal documents is essential to guide healthcare providers in delivering appropriate and respectful care.

As an Administrator, I am happy when families have representatives who advocate for the care of their loved ones. Healthcare professionals will do their best to offer respectful care in alignment with the patient's wishes; however, families know their loved ones better. Their input is encouraged and helpful.

WHAT DOES A SAMPLE HEALTHCARE POWER OF ATTORNEY FORM LOOK LIKE?

Below is a sample template for a Healthcare Power of Attorney (POA). Please note that this is a general example and may not meet the legal requirements of all states.

HEALTHCARE POWER OF ATTORNEY

I. DESIGNATION OF AGENT

I, [Your Full Name], born on [Your Date of Birth], residing at [Your Address], hereby appoint the following individual as my healthcare agent:

Agent's Name: [Agent's Full Name]

Agent's Address: [Agent's Address]

Agent's Phone Number: [Agent's Phone Number]

. . .

II. EFFECTIVE DATE

This Healthcare Power of Attorney shall become effective upon my incapacity as determined by my attending physician.

III. GRANT OF AUTHORITY

I grant my agent the authority to make any and all healthcare decisions on my behalf in accordance with my wishes, including but not limited to:

- Consent to, refuse, or withdraw consent for medical treatment, surgical procedures, medications, and any medical interventions.
- Access my medical records and obtain any information necessary to make informed decisions.
- Select and withdraw from various healthcare providers and approve referrals to specialists.
- Make decisions regarding life-sustaining treatment, including resuscitation and artificial nutrition and hydration.
- Arrange for palliative care and hospice services if indicated.

IV. ADDITIONAL INSTRUCTIONS

I wish to express the following preferences regarding my healthcare:

- [Specify any specific instructions or preferences, such as preferences for end-of-life care, organ donation, or other relevant directives.]

V. REVOCATION OF PREVIOUS DIRECTIVES
This document revokes any previous Healthcare Powers of Attorney or advance directives I may have executed.

VI. SIGNATURES

Principal's Signature:

[Your Full Name]
Date: _______________________________

VII. WITNESSES
I declare that I am not related to the principal by blood or marriage, and I am not entitled to any portion of the principal's estate upon death.

Witness 1:

[Witness's Full Name]
Address: ______________________________
Date: _______________________________

Witness 2:

[Witness's Full Name]
Address: ______________________________
Date: _______________________________

. . .

VIII. NOTARIZATION (if required by state law)

State of _____________

County of _____________

On this _____ day of _______, *20*, before me, a Notary Public, personally appeared [Your Full Name], known to me to be the person described in this instrument, and acknowledged that he/she executed the same.

Notary Public

My Commission Expires: _________________

Important Note:

- Make sure that you check with local laws, as healthcare POA requirements can vary significantly depending on the jurisdiction.
- It's advisable to discuss your wishes with your chosen agent and ensure they thoroughly understand your preferences before executing this document.
- Keep a copy of the executed document in a place where it can be easily accessed, and provide copies to your healthcare agent, family members, and healthcare providers.

You can consult with a legal professional to ensure the document fits your unique needs and complies with the laws in your state.

Skilled nursing facilities and hospitals will have templates you can utilize as well. The social service team can guide you with any additional questions.

WHAT STATES REQUIRE THE NOTARIZATION OF THE HEALTHCARE POWER OF ATTORNEY?

The requirements for notarization of a Healthcare Power of Attorney (POA) can vary significantly from state to state. While many states require a Healthcare POA to be notarized to be valid, others may accept it with just the signatures of witnesses or may have different requirements altogether. Here is a general overview:

States that Generally Require Notarization

A number of states typically require healthcare POAs to be notarized, including:

1. Alabama
2. Alaska
3. Florida
4. Georgia
5. Hawaii
6. Kentucky
7. Louisiana
8. Maryland

9. Mississippi
10. Montana
11. Nevada
12. New Hampshire
13. North Carolina
14. Ohio
15. Oklahoma
16. Tennessee
17. Texas
18. Virginia
19. Washington
20. West Virginia
21. Wisconsin

States that Do Not Require Notarization

Some states do not require notarization for a Healthcare POA but may require witness signatures instead. For example:

1. **California:** Must be signed by two witnesses unless it is notarized.
2. **New York:** Witness signatures are required; notarization is optional but advisable.
3. **Illinois:** Requires witness signatures but does not require notarization for the POA to be considered valid.

Important Notes:

- **State Laws Vary:** Always check specific state statutes or consult with a legal professional, as laws may change or may vary based on unique circumstances.

- **Best Practices:** Even if a state does not require notarization, having the document notarized can help prevent disputes and provide additional validation if the document is challenged.
- **Specific Documentation:** Some states have statutory forms with specific requirements for execution, so following those forms is crucial for validity.

Conclusion:

Consulting a lawyer or healthcare professional can ensure that state-specific guidelines are being met.

WHAT STATES REQUIRE STATUTORY FORMS FOR HEALTHCARE POWER OF ATTORNEY?

Many states in the U.S. provide statutory forms for a Healthcare Power of Attorney (POA). These forms are often included in the state's laws and are designed to meet the legal requirements for creating a valid Healthcare POA. Here are some states that have statutory forms for Healthcare Power of Attorney:

States with Statutory Forms for Healthcare Power of Attorney:

1. **California**: The state provides a statutory form for advance healthcare directives that includes a Healthcare POA.
2. **Florida**: Florida has a statutory form for designating a health care surrogate through its health care advance directives.
3. **Georgia**: Georgia provides a statutory advance directive form that combines a Healthcare POA and a living will.

4. **Hawaii**: Hawaii has a statutory form for a health care power of attorney included in its advance health care directive laws.
5. **Illinois**: Illinois provides a statutory form for a Healthcare POA within its Mental Health and Developmental Disabilities Code.
6. **Kentucky**: Kentucky has a statutory form for a healthcare surrogate designation as part of its advance directive framework.
7. **Louisiana**: Louisiana provides a statutory form known as a "Statutory Health Care Proxy" form.
8. **Maryland**: Maryland has a statutory form for an advance directive, which includes provisions for a Healthcare POA.
9. **Missouri**: Missouri offers a statutory form for a durable healthcare power of attorney.
10. **New York**: New York provides a statutory form for a Healthcare Proxy, allowing individuals to designate someone to make healthcare decisions.
11. **North Carolina**: North Carolina has a statutory form for a Health Care Power of Attorney as part of its healthcare advance directives.
12. **Ohio**: Ohio provides a statutory form for a Healthcare POA within its advance directives law.
13. **Pennsylvania**: Pennsylvania provides a statutory form for a Health Care Power of Attorney as part of its health care advance directive law.
14. **South Carolina**: South Carolina has a statutory form for a Health Care Power of Attorney included in its advance directives.
15. **Texas**: Texas has a statutory form for a Medical Power of Attorney as part of its healthcare advance directives.

16. **Virginia**: Virginia provides a statutory form for a Medical Power of Attorney that allows an individual to appoint an agent for health care purposes.
17. **Washington**: Washington offers a statutory advance directive form, which includes a healthcare power of attorney.
18. **West Virginia**: West Virginia has a statutory form for a Health Care Power of Attorney as part of its state code.

Important Considerations:

- **Consultation**: It is essential to read and understand the statutory form provided by your state and consult with a legal professional if you have specific questions or unique circumstances.
- **Accessibility**: Most state government websites or legal aid organizations provide access to these statutory forms, often in downloadable PDF format.

Conclusion:

Statutory forms can provide clarity and ensure compliance with state requirements when creating a Healthcare Power of Attorney. Always ensure that you fill out the form correctly and consider discussing your healthcare wishes with your appointed agent and any family members involved.

WHAT DO HEALTHCARE PROFESSIONALS DO IF THERE IS NO SURROGATE DECISION MAKER OR HEALTHCARE POWER OF ATTORNEY SET UP?

When there is no surrogate decision-maker or Healthcare Power of Attorney (POA) in place, healthcare workers face a challenging situation when it comes to making medical decisions for a patient who is unable to communicate their wishes due to incapacity. In such cases, healthcare professionals typically follow certain protocols and guidelines to ensure that appropriate care is provided. Here are the actions they may take:

1. Follow State Laws and Regulations:

- Healthcare providers must adhere to the laws of the state regarding decision-making for incapacitated patients. Many states have statutes outlining a hierarchy of individuals who can serve as surrogate decision-makers, even in the absence of a formal Healthcare POA.

2. Consult the Patient's Family:

- If no POA exists, healthcare workers may reach out to the patient's family members or close friends to understand the patient's values, preferences, and possible wishes regarding treatment. Family members may often be given priority in decision-making roles according to state laws.

3. Use of a Medical Ethics Committee:

- Some healthcare facilities have medical ethics committees that can guide in situations where there is uncertainty about patient care decisions in the absence of an agent. These committees can help mediate disputes and ensure that the patient's best interests are considered.

4. Assessing the Patient's Wishes:

- Healthcare providers should document any known patient preferences, values, or previously expressed wishes, even if not formally documented. This may be gleaned from family discussions, previous medical records, or informal communications.

5. Act in the Best Interest of the Patient:

- In the absence of clear directives from the patient, healthcare workers are often guided by the principle of acting in the patient's best interest. This may involve evaluating the potential benefits, risks, and burdens of proposed treatments and making decisions that align with what is typically considered reasonable and ethical care for similar patients.

6. Seek Court Intervention:

- If necessary, healthcare workers may consider seeking legal intervention to appoint a temporary guardian or conservator for the patient. This process may involve obtaining a court order to determine who can make healthcare decisions on the patient's behalf.

7. Emergency Situations:

- In emergency situations where immediate decisions need to be made, and no surrogate is available, medical professionals are typically empowered to provide necessary treatment based on standard medical practices to stabilize the patient.

8. Documentation:

- Healthcare workers should document all decisions, discussions, and attempts to contact family members or seek surrogate involvement. Clear documentation is crucial for legal and ethical accountability.

Conclusion:

Healthcare workers must navigate complex legal and ethical considerations when faced with incapacitated patients who lack designated decision-makers. Establishing advance directives, such as a Healthcare Power of Attorney, is critical for ensuring that medical decisions reflect patients' wishes and values. Healthcare institutions encourage individuals to create these documents to facilitate better decision-making in advance of potential incapacity.

Further in this book, Guardianship will be covered in detail; however, now we will cover additional forms of power of attorney.

WHAT IS FINANCIAL POWER OF ATTORNEY?

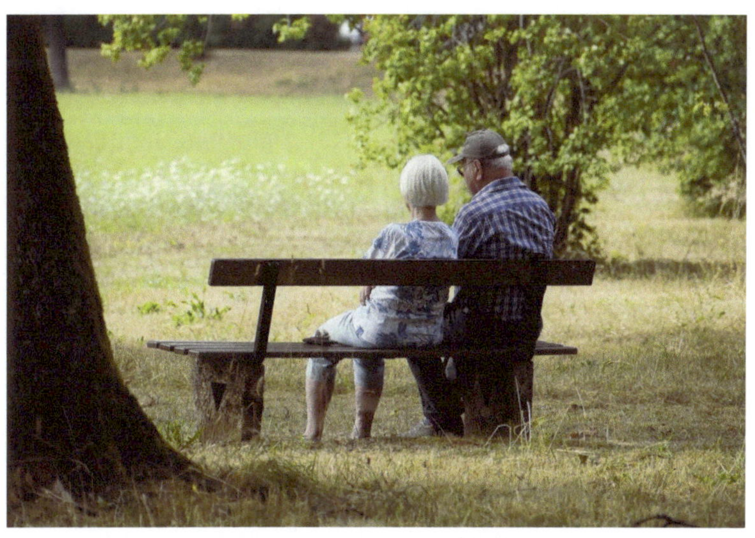

A financial power of Attorney (POA) is a legal document that allows an individual (the principal) to designate another person (the agent or attorney-in-fact) to manage their financial affairs and make financial decisions on their behalf. This type of POA can be general or limited in scope, depending on the principal's needs and preferences.

Key Features of Financial Power of Attorney:

1. **Authority Granted:** A Financial Power of Attorney can grant the agent a variety of powers, including but not limited to:
   - Managing bank accounts (e.g., depositing, withdrawing, transferring funds).
   - Paying bills, debts, and expenses.
   - Filing tax returns and handling tax matters.
   - Managing investments, real estate transactions, and financial assets.
   - Making decisions about insurance policies.
   - Managing retirement accounts and pensions.
   - Signing documents related to financial transactions.
2. **Types of Financial POA:**
   - General Financial Power of Attorney: Gives the agent broad authority to act on behalf of the principal in a wide range of financial matters.
   - Limited Financial Power of Attorney: Restricts the agent's authority to specific tasks or for a defined period. For example, it may only allow the agent to sell a particular piece of property or manage financial affairs while the principal is traveling.

3. **Durability:** A Financial Power of Attorney can be either durable or non-durable. A durable financial POA remains in effect even if the principal becomes incapacitated, while a non-durable POA becomes invalid upon the principal's incapacitation.
4. **Revocation:** The principal can revoke a Financial Power of Attorney at any time, as long as they are mentally competent. This revocation should be documented in writing, and copies should be provided to the agent and any relevant institutions.
5. **Execution Requirements:** To be valid, a Financial Power of Attorney must typically meet certain legal requirements, which may include:
    - Signature of the principal.
    - Witnesses (varies by state).
    - Notarization (often required in many states).
6. **Choosing an Agent:** The principal should choose someone trustworthy and capable of handling financial matters as their agent. This person may be a family member, friend, or professional, such as an attorney or financial advisor.

Importance of Financial Power of Attorney:

Having a Financial POA in place is crucial for individuals who may need assistance managing their financial affairs due to incapacity or other reasons. It ensures that someone they trust can act in their best interest and manage their financial responsibilities without delay.

Conclusion:

Creating a Financial Power of Attorney can help provide

peace of mind regarding financial management, particularly for seniors or individuals with health concerns. It is advisable to consult with a legal professional when drafting this document to ensure it meets all legal requirements and accurately reflects the principal's intentions regarding their financial affairs.

WHAT FORMS ARE NEEDED FOR FINANCIAL POWER OF ATTORNEY?

To create a Financial Power of Attorney (POA), specific forms and documentation are generally required. While the exact requirements can vary by state, the following components are commonly needed:

1. Financial Power of Attorney Document:

- This is the primary form that outlines the authority granted to the agent (attorney-in-fact). The document should include:
  - The names and contact information of the principal (the person granting the power) and the agent (the person receiving the power).
  - A clear statement that this is a Financial Power of Attorney.
  - The specific powers granted to the agent may include managing bank accounts, paying bills, selling or managing property, handling investment decisions, and any other financial matters.

- Whether the POA is general or limited, and if limited, the specific tasks for which the agent is authorized.
- Indication of whether the POA is durable (remaining in effect if the principal becomes incapacitated) or non-durable.
- Any limitations or restrictions on the authority of the agent.
- The effective date of the POA (immediate or upon the occurrence of a specific event).

2. Signatures:

- The principal must sign the Financial Power of Attorney document. Depending on state laws, the agent may also need to sign to acknowledge acceptance of the role.

3. Witnesses:

- Most states require that the Financial Power of Attorney be signed in the presence of one or more witnesses. The number of witnesses may vary by state, so it's important to check local laws.

4. Notarization:

- Many states require the Financial Power of Attorney to be notarized to be considered valid. A notary public must witness the signing of the document and affix their seal to it.

5. State-Specific Requirements:

- It is crucial to review the specific laws for your state because each state may have unique requirements or statutory forms for Financial Powers of Attorney.

6. Distribution of Copies:

- After the Financial Power of Attorney is executed, it is recommended to provide copies to:
    - The agent who is named in the document.
    - Financial institutions (e.g., banks, investment firms) where the principal has accounts, so they are aware of the agent's authority.
    - Family members or other relevant parties as needed.

Conclusion:

While templates for Financial Power of Attorney forms are often available online, it is highly advisable to consult with a legal professional to ensure that the document meets all legal requirements and adequately reflects the principal's wishes. This helps prevent issues or misunderstandings regarding the authority granted to the agent.

In healthcare settings such as skilled nursing, healthcare professionals cannot help determine financial powers of attorney. In fact, if there is no one to manage a resident's funds, state guardianship may need to be set up, as healthcare professionals cannot manage a resident's or patient's funds. In skilled nursing settings, there is usually a business office manager who can set up a trust fund, which is like a bank account, but we are not managing the resident's funds; we are only helping facilitate payment like a bank account.

WHAT IS REVOCATION OF POWER OF ATTORNEY?

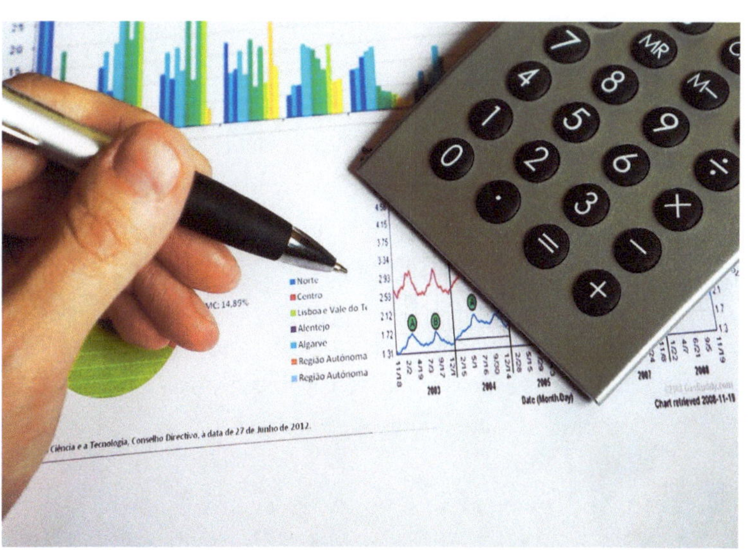

Revocation of Power of Attorney is the formal process by which a principal (the person who created the Power of Attorney) terminates the authority granted to an agent (the person designated to act on the principal's behalf). This revocation can occur for various reasons, including changes in circumstances, loss of trust in the agent, or the principal's change of mind. Here are the key aspects of revoking a Power of Attorney:

Key Features of Revocation of Power of Attorney:

1. **Written Notice**:
   - The principal must typically create a written document stating that the Power of Attorney is being revoked. This document is often referred to as a "Revocation of Power of Attorney."
   - The revocation notice should clearly identify the original Power of Attorney by mentioning the date it was executed and the names of the principal and the agent.
2. **Signatures**:
   - The principal must sign the revocation document. In some cases, witnesses or notarization may be required, depending on state laws.
3. **Notification**:
   - The principal must notify the agent that their authority has been revoked. This can prevent the agent from inadvertently making decisions in the principal's name after the revocation.
   - Additionally, it's important to notify any third parties (such as banks or medical providers) who may have relied on the original Power of Attorney that the agent's authority has been revoked.

4. **Effective Date**:
   - The revocation generally becomes effective as soon as it is executed and delivered to the agent and relevant third parties unless specified otherwise in the revocation document.
5. **Creating a New Power of Attorney**:
   - If the principal wants to appoint a new agent or make changes to the powers granted, they can create a new Power of Attorney. It is essential to ensure that the new document explicitly revokes any previous powers to avoid confusion.
6. **Legal Capacity**:
   - The principal must be mentally competent to revoke a Power of Attorney. If the principal becomes incapacitated, they typically cannot revoke the Power of Attorney, and the authority granted may continue until the principal's death or until a court intervenes.
7. **Implications for the Agent**:
   - Once a Power of Attorney is revoked, the former agent no longer has the legal authority to act on behalf of the principal. Any actions or decisions made by the agent after the revocation are unauthorized and may be considered invalid.

Importance of Revocation:

Revocation of Power of Attorney is a critical mechanism that allows individuals to maintain control over their legal and financial affairs. It provides a way to change agents or modify their powers as personal circumstances change. It also ensures that individuals can refresh their plans and address any changes in trust or preferences.

Conclusion:

If a principal decides to revoke a Power of Attorney. In that case, it is advisable to consult with a legal professional to ensure the revocation is executed properly and in accordance with state laws and to minimize the risk of misunderstandings or disputes.

WHAT FORMS ARE NEEDED FOR REVOCATION OF POWER OF ATTORNEY?

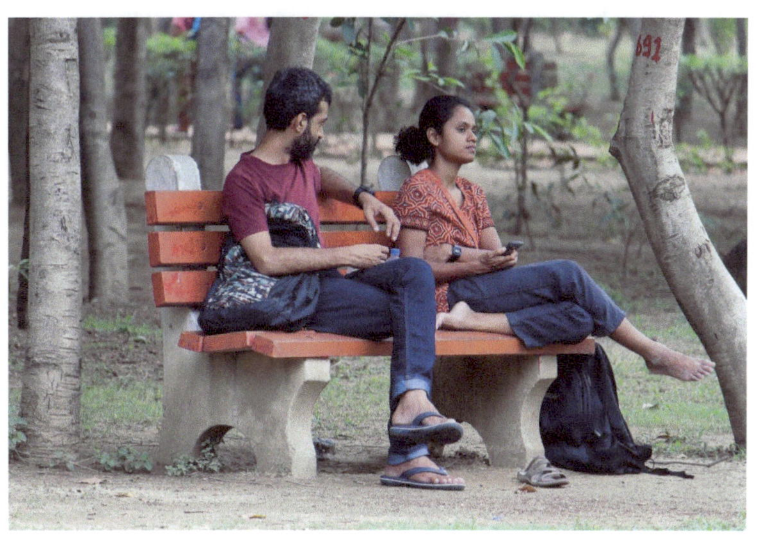

To revoke a Power of Attorney (POA), specific forms and procedures need to be followed to ensure that the revocation is legally valid and recognized. Here are the necessary components typically involved in the revocation process:

1. Revocation of Power of Attorney Document:

- A written document specifically stating that the existing Power of Attorney is being revoked. This document should include:
    - The title "Revocation of Power of Attorney" should be at the top.
    - The date the revocation is executed.
    - The names of the principal and the agent whose authority is being revoked.
    - A reference to the original Power of Attorney document (e.g., the date it was signed).
    - A clear statement that the principal revokes all powers granted to the agent.
    - The signature of the principal.

Sample Format:

text

REVOCATION OF POWER OF ATTORNEY

I, [Your Full Name], born on [Your Date of Birth], residing at [Your Address], hereby revoke the Power of Attorney executed on [Date of Original POA], in which I appointed [Agent's Name] as my agent.

This revocation is effective immediately upon execution.

Principal's Signature: _________________________________

Date: _______________________________

2. Signatures:

- The principal must sign the revocation document. Depending on state laws, the document may also need to be witnessed or notarized.

3. Witnesses and Notarization:

- Many states require that the revocation document be either witnessed or notarized. It's important to check state-specific requirements regarding signatures and verification.

4. Notification:

- Although not a formal "form," it is essential to notify the previously appointed agent of the revocation. This can often be done through a simple letter or email.
- Additionally, the principal should notify any relevant institutions (such as banks, healthcare providers, etc.) that may have relied on the original Power of Attorney.

5. Distribution of Copies:

- After completing the revocation, it's important to provide copies of the revocation document to:
    - The revoked agent.
    - All institutions and individuals that were aware of the original Power of Attorney.
    - Personal records.

Conclusion:

While templates for the Revocation of Power of Attorney can often be found online, it is advisable to consult with a legal professional to ensure that the document meets all legal requirements specific to your state and adequately reflects your intentions. Proper execution and notification will help to prevent any future misunderstandings regarding the agent's authority.

From a healthcare professional perspective, it is very helpful to have a surrogate or power of attorney clearly selected.

In my time as an Administrator, there have been several times where there was more than one power of attorney. The most recent forms of power of attorney are the ones that take validity over the others. Also, if there are state-specific requirements, if one document has the requirements and one does not, the form with the state-specific requirements will take precedence. If a state-appointed Guardian is in place, that person takes authority over the written powers of attorney. This can happen in elderly abuse cases.

GUARDIANSHIP

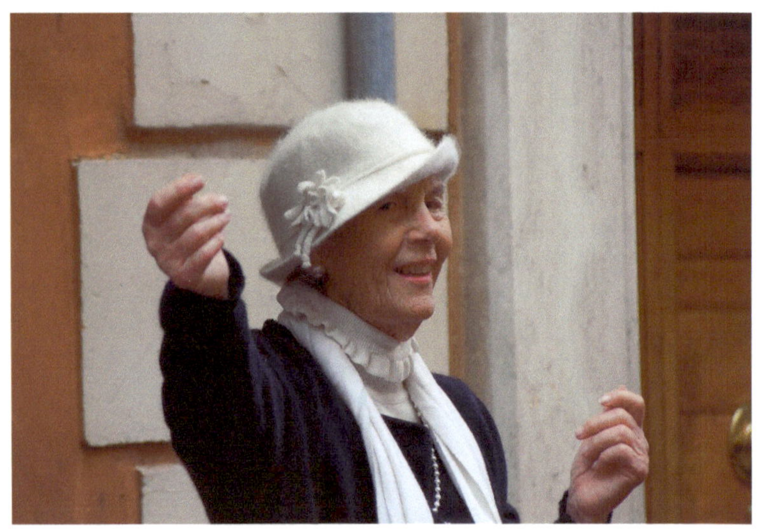

This is a great segway into talking about Guardianship.

Guardianship is a legal relationship established by a court in which one person (the guardian) is appointed to make decisions on behalf of another person (the ward) who is unable to make those decisions due to incapacity, disability, or minors (children under a certain age). The purpose of guardianship is to protect the interests and welfare of individuals who cannot manage their personal, financial, or medical affairs.

Key Aspects of Guardianship:

1. **Types of Guardianship**:
   - **Guardianship of the Person**: Provides the guardian with the authority to make personal decisions for the ward, which may include decisions about living arrangements, education, medical care, and overall welfare.
   - **Guardianship of the Estate**: Grants the guardian authority over the ward's financial matters, including managing financial assets, paying bills, and making investment decisions.
   - **Combination Guardianship**: A guardian may be appointed for both personal and financial matters.
2. **Court Involvement**:
   - Guardianship is typically established through a legal process in court. A petition must be filed by concerned parties (which could include family members, friends, or social services) to have a guardian appointed. The court will assess the alleged incapacity of the individual (the ward) and determine whether guardianship is appropriate.
3. **Criteria for Appointment**:
   - The individual being considered for guardianship must demonstrate an inability to manage their personal or financial affairs due to mental

incapacity, developmental disability, substance abuse, or being a minor.
- Courts require evidence or assessments from medical professionals to support the claim of incapacity.

4. **Responsibilities of the Guardian**:
   - A guardian has a fiduciary duty to act in the best interests of the ward and to manage their affairs responsibly. Responsibilities can include:
     - Making healthcare decisions consistent with the ward's best interests and known wishes.
     - Managing and protecting the ward's financial resources.
     - Keeping accurate records of all decisions made and transactions performed on behalf of the ward.
     - Reporting to the court regarding the ward's condition and the guardianship's management, as required.

5. **Duration of Guardianship**:
   - Guardianship can be temporary or permanent, depending on the needs of the ward and the reasons for the guardianship. Temporary guardianship may be granted for a limited time (for example, during a medical emergency).

6. **Termination of Guardianship**:
   - Guardianship can be terminated if the ward regains capacity, if the guardian fails to fulfill their duties, or if circumstances change that warrant a different arrangement.
   - A petition for termination can be filed in court by the guardian or another interested party.

7. **Alternatives to Guardianship**:

○ In some cases, individuals may choose alternatives to guardianship, such as powers of attorney, advance healthcare directives, or supported decision-making agreements, allowing individuals to retain some level of autonomy while receiving assistance.

Conclusion:

Guardianship is a critical legal tool designed to protect individuals who are unable to make decisions for themselves. It involves significant responsibilities for the guardian and oversight by the court, ensuring that the ward's best interests are prioritized. If guardianship is being considered for a loved one, it is advisable to consult with a legal professional experienced in elder law or family law for guidance and assistance through the court process.

A high-profile case of guardianship that was in the news was that of Britney Spears, where her father had control of her financial affairs through guardianship. Britney Spears fought and won to have this revoked. Guardianship can be active for anyone of any age. Through the process, it is determined that the ward cannot manage their own person or finances.

In skilled nursing settings, if there are no surrogate decision makers or power of attorney in place and the person is incapable of managing their person or finances, the facility may petition for a state guardian to oversee them. As was mentioned earlier, there are several medical situations in which healthcare personnel cannot make decisions for the resident. Also, in some cases, where there is an abusive family member associated with a person needing medical care, a state guardian will be appointed.

HOW DO YOU ATTAIN GUARDIANSHIP FOR AN INDIVIDUAL?

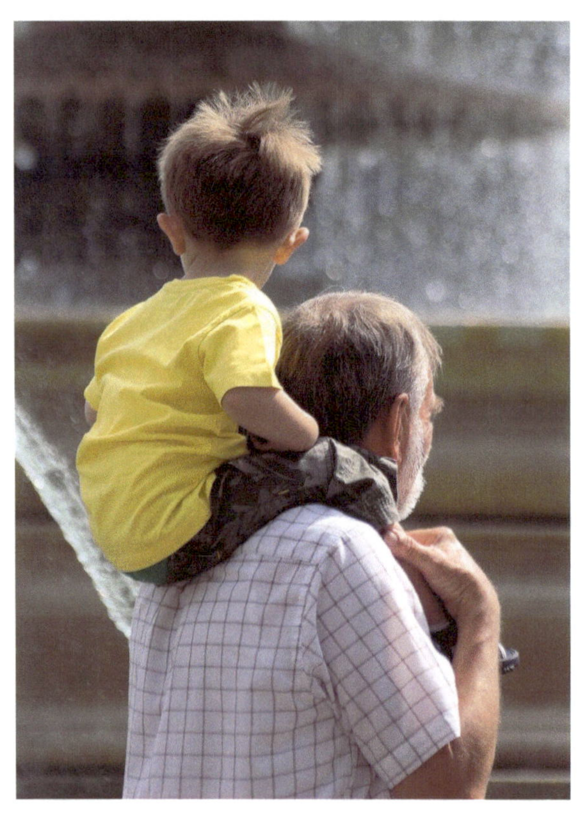

Attaining guardianship for an individual involves a legal process, typically requiring court approval. The specific steps may vary by state or jurisdiction, but the general process usually includes the following steps:

Steps to Attain Guardianship:

1. **Determine the Need for Guardianship**:
   - Assess whether the individual (the potential ward) is unable to make decisions regarding their personal, medical, or financial affairs due to incapacitation, disability, age (if a minor), or other reasons.
2. **Research State Laws**:
   - Review the guardianship laws specific to your state or jurisdiction. Each state has its statutes and processes for establishing guardianship, including forms, filing fees, and requirements for those requesting guardianship.
3. **File a Petition**:
   - Complete and file a petition for guardianship with the appropriate court. This petition typically includes:
     - Information about the petitioner (the person seeking guardianship).
     - Information about the alleged incapacitated individual (the ward).
     - Reasons for requesting guardianship, including evidence of incapacity.
     - An explanation of the type of guardianship being sought (guardian of the person, guardian of the estate, or both).

     ○ The petition may also require supporting documents, such as medical evaluations or assessments, to establish the need for guardianship.

4. **Notify Interested Parties**:
     ○ In most cases, the petitioner must provide notice of the guardianship proceedings to interested parties, including:
        ■ The individual for whom guardianship is requested.
        ■ Immediate family members.
     ○ Depending on state laws, you may need to file proof of service with the court.

5. **Attend the Court Hearing**:
     ○ A court hearing will be scheduled where the petitioner must present evidence to demonstrate the necessity for guardianship. This may include:
        ■ Testimony from medical professionals regarding the ward's capacity.
        ■ Statements from family members or others familiar with the situation.
     ○ The alleged incapacitated individual may also be involved in the hearing to express their views, if possible.

6. **Court Decision**:
     ○ After reviewing the evidence and testimony, the court will make a decision regarding the appointment of guardianship. If granted, the court will issue a guardianship order specifying the powers and responsibilities of the guardian.

7. **Obtain Letters of Guardianship**:
     ○ If the court grants guardianship, the guardian will receive legal documents (letters of guardianship or guardianship certificate) that authorize them to

act on behalf of the ward. These documents may be required when dealing with third parties (e.g., banks, healthcare providers).

8. **Fulfill Ongoing Responsibilities**:
   - The guardian is required to fulfill their duties as outlined by the court, which may include:
     - Making decisions in the best interests of the ward.
     - Keeping records of the ward's finances and health care decisions.
     - Reporting to the court, if required, about the ward's condition or the guardian's actions.

9. **Review and Termination**:
   - Guardianship may be reviewed periodically by the court to ensure that it is still necessary. Guardianship can also be terminated if the ward regains capacity or if circumstances change, such as the guardian failing to act in the ward's best interest.

Conclusion:

Attaining guardianship is a significant legal undertaking that requires careful consideration, documentation, and compliance with legal procedures. It is advisable to consult with an attorney knowledgeable in guardianship or family law to ensure that the process is followed correctly and to navigate any complexities that may arise. This legal support can help clarify duties, responsibilities, and the rights of both the guardian and the ward throughout the guardianship process.

HOW MUCH DOES IT COST TO ATTAIN GUARDIANSHIP OF AN INDIVIDUAL?

The cost of attaining guardianship of an individual can vary widely based on several factors, including the complexity of the case, the state or jurisdiction, and whether legal assistance is needed. Here are some key components that contribute to the overall cost:

1. Court Filing Fees:

- Each state has its own set of filing fees associated with the guardianship petition. These fees can range from **$50 to $400** or more, depending on the court and the specific filings required.

2. Legal Fees:

- If you choose to hire an attorney to assist with the guardianship process, legal fees will be one of the most significant costs. Attorneys may charge a flat fee for guardianship cases or bill by the hour, with rates typically ranging from **$150 to $500 per hour**.

- Flat fees for a straightforward guardianship case can range from **$1,000 to $4,000** or higher, especially if the case involves complex issues, disputes among family members, or the need for extensive legal documentation.

3. Costs for Medical Evaluations:

- In many cases, a medical evaluation or assessment may be required to determine the alleged incapacitated individual's ability to make decisions. This may involve fees for healthcare professionals to conduct evaluations, which can range from **$100 to $500** or more.

4. Cost of Process Servers:

- If you need to serve notice to interested parties or family members, you may incur additional expenses for process servers, which can range from **$25 to $100** or more, depending on the service required.

5. Miscellaneous Costs:

- There may be additional costs for copy services, documentation preparation, postage, or other administrative expenses.

6. Ongoing Costs:

- Once guardianship is established, there may be ongoing costs for guardianship administration, including yearly reports to the court, accounting for the ward's finances, and possible legal fees if disputes arise.

Summary of Costs:

- **Court Filing Fees**: $50 to $400+
- **Legal Fees**: $1,000 to $4,000+ (or hourly rates of $150 to $500)
- **Medical Evaluations**: $100 to $500+
- **Process Servers**: $25 to $100+
- **Miscellaneous Costs**: Variable

Conclusion

Overall, the total cost to attain guardianship of an individual can range from **a few hundred dollars to several thousand dollars**, depending on the complexity and specifics of the case. It is advisable to consult with a legal professional to get a clearer estimate based on your unique situation and needs. Additionally, checking with local courts for specific fee schedules and potential fee waivers for low-income applicants can also be beneficial.

FOR EXAMPLE, IN THE STATE OF ILLINOIS, WHAT WEBSITE DO YOU VISIT TO START THE GUARDIANSHIP PROCESS?

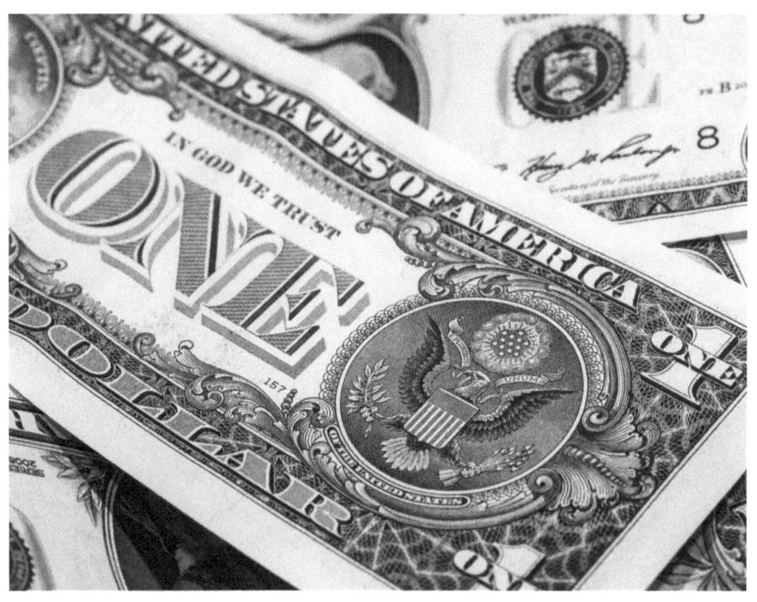

In Illinois, the guardianship process is primarily handled through the circuit court in the county where the individual for whom guardianship is being sought resides. To start the guardianship process and access the necessary forms and information, you can visit the **Illinois Courts** website.

The following are the relevant resources where you can find information about starting the guardianship process in Illinois:

1. Illinois Courts Website:

- The official website of the Illinois Courts provides general information on guardianship and links to necessary forms:
- Illinois Courts Guardianship Information: https://www.illinoiscourts.gov

2. Illinois Department of Healthcare and Family Services:

- For additional resources and guidelines related to guardianship, including links to forms, the Illinois Department of Healthcare and Family Services has information that can be helpful:
- Illinois Healthcare and Family Services: https://hfs.illinois.gov/

3. Illinois Guardianship and Advocacy Commission

- Illinois Guardianship and Advocacy Commission has a lot of great resources and information about guardianship in relation to protecting those with disabilities.

- Illinois Guardianship and Advocacy Commission: https://gac.illinois.gov/

4. Local Circuit Court Website:

- You should also consult the website of the circuit court in your specific county, as each county may have its own rules, forms, and procedures regarding guardianship. You can typically find forms and local procedures by searching for "Circuit Court [Your County Name] Illinois" online.

Example for Cook County:

If you are in Cook County, you can visit the Cook County Circuit Court website for guardianship forms and specific instructions:

- Cook County Circuit Court Guardianship: https://www.cookcountycourt.org

Conclusion:

Using the Illinois Courts website and your local circuit court's website, you can access the necessary information, forms, and guidelines to initiate the guardianship process in Illinois. If you have further questions or need assistance, it can also be beneficial to consult with an attorney who specializes in guardianship or family law in Illinois.

FOR EXAMPLE, IN THE STATE OF FLORIDA, WHAT WEBSITE DO YOU VISIT TO START THE GUARDIANSHIP PROCESS?

In Florida, you can start the guardianship process by visiting the official website of the **Florida State Courts**. They provide comprehensive information regarding guardianship, including necessary forms and procedures. Here are the relevant resources:

1. Florida State Courts Website:

- The Florida State Courts website includes detailed information about guardianship proceedings and links to the appropriate forms:
- Florida State Courts - Guardianship: https://www.flcourts.gov/Resources-Services/Office-of-Family-Courts/Family-Court-in-Florida/Guardianship

2. Local Circuit Court Websites:

- Since guardianship is handled at the local circuit court level, you should also check the website of your specific circuit court. Each county may have its own rules and requirements for guardianship proceedings.

- You can find your local circuit court website by searching for "Circuit Court [Your County] Florida" online.

Example for Miami-Dade County:

If you are in Miami-Dade County, you can go directly to their court's website for guardianship-related resources:

- Miami-Dade County Circuit Court Guardianship: https://www.miami-dadeclerk.com

Additional Resources:

- **Florida Department of Elder Affairs**: The Florida Department of Elder Affairs also has resources regarding guardianship and other elder law issues. Their website can provide valuable information:
  - Florida Department of Elder Affairs: https://elderaffairs.org

Conclusion:

Using the Florida State Courts website and your local circuit court's website, you can access the necessary information and forms to initiate the guardianship process in Florida. If you have specific questions or require legal assistance, it may also be beneficial to consult an attorney specializing in guardianship and family law in Florida.

FOR EXAMPLE, IN THE STATE OF CALIFORNIA, WHAT WEBSITE DO YOU VISIT TO START THE GUARDIANSHIP PROCESS?

In California, you can start the guardianship process by visiting the California Courts website, which provides resources and information regarding guardianship proceedings, including necessary forms and procedures. Here are the relevant resources:

1. California Courts Website:

- The California Courts website has a section specifically dedicated to guardianships, outlining the process, requirements, and links to necessary forms:
- California Courts - Guardianship: https://selfhelp. courts.ca.gov/guardianship

2. Instructions and Forms:

- You can find detailed instructions on how to complete the guardianship process, including court forms:
- California Guardianship Forms: https://www.courts.

ca.gov/partners/documents/permanent_guardian
ship_forms.pdf

3. Local Superior Court Websites:

- Guardianship cases are filed in the local Superior Court. You should also check the website of your specific county's Superior Court for local procedures and additional resources. To find your county's court information, you can use the following link:
- California Superior Courts: https://www.courts.ca. gov/find-my-court.htm

Example for Los Angeles County:

If you are in Los Angeles County, you can directly visit the Los Angeles Superior Court's website for more information about guardianship:

- Los Angeles County Superior Court - Guardianship: https://www.lacourt.org

4. California Department of Social Services:

- The California Department of Social Services provides additional resources related to guardianship, especially concerning the welfare of children:
- California Department of Social Services: https:// www.cdss.ca.gov

Conclusion:

By visiting the California Courts website and your local Superior Court's website, you can access the necessary information and forms to initiate the guardianship process in California. If you have specific questions or complexities in your case, consulting an attorney who specializes in guardianship or family law may be beneficial.

IN THE STATE OF NEW YORK, WHAT WEBSITES DO YOU VISIT TO START THE GUARDIANSHIP PROCESS?

I n New York, you can start the guardianship process by visiting the New York State Unified Court System's website, which provides comprehensive information about the guardianship process, including necessary forms and procedures. Here are the relevant resources:

1. New York State Unified Court System Website:

- The official website offers guidance on guardianships, including procedures for both guardianship of the person and guardianship of the property:
- New York State Unified Court System - Guardianship: https://www.nycourts.gov/courthelp/ Guardianship/guardianship.shtml

2. Guardianship Forms:

- You can find and download the required forms to initiate a guardianship application. The website provides instructions along with links to the necessary forms:

- New York Court Forms: https://www.nycourts.gov/forms/

3. Local County Court Websites:

- The guardianship process is handled at the county level. You should also check the website of your specific county court for local procedures, additional resources, and any county-specific forms. To find your local court, you can access:
- Find My Court: https://www.nycourts.gov/courts/

Example for New York County (Manhattan):

If you are in Manhattan (New York County), you can directly visit the New York County Supreme Court website for guardianship information:

- New York County Supreme Court - Guardianship: https://www.nycourts.gov/courts/1jd/supreme/nyc/index.shtml

Additional Resources:

- The New York State Office of Children and Family Services also provides information on guardianship, especially related to child guardianship, which can be found on their website:
- New York State Office of Children and Family Services: https://ocfs.ny.gov/main/

Conclusion:

By visiting the New York State Unified Court System website and the specific county court website, you can access the necessary information and forms to initiate the guardianship process in New York. If you encounter specific questions or complexities in your case, consulting an attorney who specializes in family law or guardianship may be beneficial.

IN THE STATE OF TEXAS, WHAT WEBSITES DO YOU VISIT TO START THE GUARDIANSHIP PROCESS?

In the state of Texas, you can begin the guardianship process by visiting the Texas Judicial Branch's official website, which provides information about guardianship, the legal process involved, and the necessary forms. Here are the relevant resources:

1. Texas Judicial Branch Website:

- The Texas Judicial Branch offers information on guardianship, including links to forms and instructions for the process:
  - **Texas Guardianship Information: https://www. txcourts.gov/**

2. Local County Court Websites:

- Guardianship cases are managed at the local level in Texas counties. It's important to check the website of your specific county's probate or district court for

specific procedures, local forms, and additional resources. You can find your local court by visiting:
- ○ **Find My Court**

Example for Harris County:

If you are in Harris County (Houston), you can visit the Harris County Probate Court website for guardianship information:

- **Harris County Probate Court: https://probate. harriscountytx.gov/**

3. Texas Health and Human Services

- Texas health and human services website outlines the guardianship process and offers helpful information
- Texas Health and Human Services: https://www.hhs. texas.gov/regulations/legal-information/guardianship

Additional Resources:

- The Texas Guardianship Association also provides valuable information about guardianship laws and resources in Texas:
  - ○ **Texas Guardianship Association: https://www. txguardian.com**

Conclusion:

By visiting the Texas Judicial Branch website, accessing the required forms, and checking your local county court's website, you can initiate the guardianship process in Texas. If you have specific questions or need legal assistance, it may be helpful to consult with an attorney who specializes in guardianship or family law in Texas.

Every state has a set of court system websites that can be visited to review the specific Guardianship forms and procedures.

What Are All of the Circumstances That Would Warrant Guardianship?

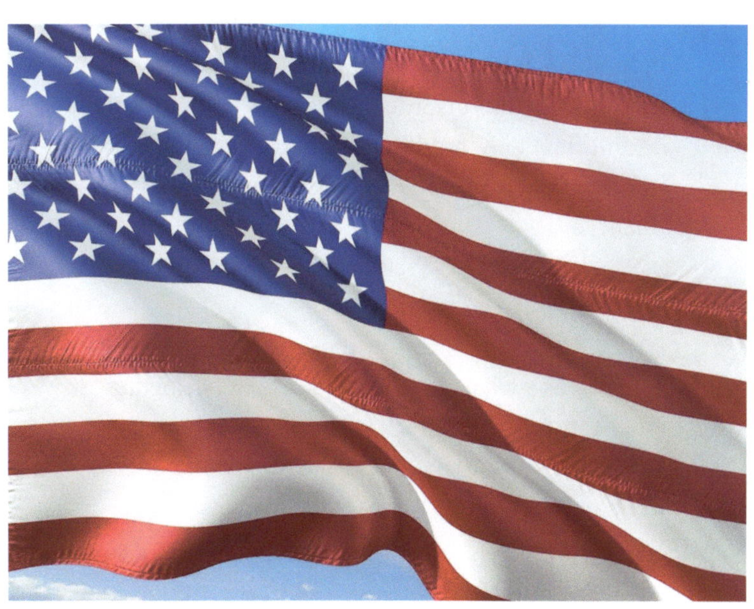

Guardianship is a legal arrangement established to protect individuals who are unable to make decisions for themselves due to various circumstances. Here are the common situations that may warrant establishing a guardianship:

1. Incapacity Due to Mental Illness:

- Individuals suffering from mental health conditions that significantly impair their decision-making ability may need a guardian to manage their personal and/or financial affairs.

2. Developmental Disabilities:

- Individuals with developmental disabilities (such as autism spectrum disorders or intellectual disabilities) may not have the capacity to make informed decisions about their personal care or finances.

3. Severe Cognitive Impairment:

- Conditions such as Alzheimer's disease, dementia, or other forms of cognitive impairment can limit an individual's ability to understand and communicate decisions regarding their care or finances.

4. Substance Abuse:

- Individuals struggling with substance abuse issues may be unable to make sound decisions regarding their health, safety, and finances, thereby necessitating guardianship.

5. Age-Related Decline:

- Older adults may face diminished capacity due to age-related conditions, which can affect their cognitive abilities, thereby potentially making them candidates for guardianship.

6. Physical Disability:

- Severe physical disabilities that limit an individual's ability to care for themselves and manage their affairs might require a guardian to ensure their needs are met.

7. Minor Children:

- Minors who do not have a natural guardian (such as a deceased or unfit parent) might require a guardian to manage their personal and financial matters until they reach adulthood.

8. Temporary Incapacity:

- Situations such as severe illness, recovery from surgery, or temporary incapacitating conditions (e.g., coma) may lead to a request for temporary guardianship to make short-term decisions on behalf of the incapacitated person.

9. Inability to Manage Finances:

- Adults who cannot manage their financial affairs due to cognitive impairment, addiction, or other mental health issues may warrant guardianship, particularly to prevent exploitation or mismanagement of finances.

10. Legal Issues:

- In some cases, individuals facing legal difficulties (e.g., incarceration or involvement in the criminal justice system) may require guardianship for certain decisions while they are unable to make those decisions themselves.

Conclusion:

Guardianship is a serious legal measure designed to protect those who genuinely cannot manage their own affairs. Establishing guardianship typically requires a court process to evaluate the necessity and appropriateness of such a protective arrangement. It is essential to approach guardianship carefully, considering all alternatives, such as powers of attorney or supported decision-making agreements, which may empower individuals while allowing for necessary support. Consulting with a legal professional experienced in guardianship can provide further guidance in navigating these complex issues.

WHEN WOULD GUARDIANSHIP BE DENIED?

A court may deny guardianship for a variety of reasons. The decision depends on the evidence presented and the specific legal standards in each jurisdiction. Here are common reasons that could lead to the denial of a guardianship application:

1. Lack of Incapacity:

- If the court determines that the individual (the proposed ward) is still capable of making informed decisions regarding their personal affairs, guardianship will typically be denied. This can occur if:
  - The proposed ward can understand the nature of their situation and make decisions.
  - Evidence or testimonies from medical professionals indicate that the individual is competent.

2. Unclear Evidence of Need:

- If the petitioner fails to provide compelling evidence that the proposed ward needs a guardian, the court may deny the application. This includes a lack of:
  - Medical evaluations supporting claims of incapacity.
  - Clear documentation of the individual's inability to manage their affairs.

3. Improper Procedure:

- Guardianship applications must comply with specific legal procedures and requirements. If the petitioner fails to follow these processes, the court may dismiss the case. This can include:
  - Not providing proper notices to interested parties.
  - Failing to file the appropriate forms or documents.

4. Choice of Guardian:

- The court may deny guardianship if the proposed guardian does not meet the legal qualifications or if there are concerns about their ability to serve in the role. Reasons may include:
  - A history of financial mismanagement or criminal behavior.
  - A conflict of interest or inability to act in the best interest of the ward.

5. Less Restrictive Alternatives Available:

- If there are less restrictive alternatives to guardianship that can adequately meet the needs of the individual (e.g., powers of attorney, healthcare directives, or supported decision-making arrangements). In that case, the court may deny the petition for guardianship.

6. Competent and Suitable Alternatives:

- If other family members or parties are willing and able to provide support or care without the need for formal guardianship, the court may decline to grant guardianship to the petitioner.

7. Potential for Abuse or Misuse of Power:

- If there is reasonable concern that the proposed guardian may misuse their authority or fail to act in the best interest of the proposed ward, the court may deny guardianship. This includes:
  - Evidence of prior abuse, neglect, or exploitation.

8. Family Conflict:

- If there are significant disputes or conflicts among family members regarding the need for guardianship or the choice of guardian. In that case, the court may choose not to establish guardianship until these issues are resolved.

Conclusion:

The denial of a guardianship application typically reflects the court's commitment to ensuring that individuals are only placed under guardianship when it is genuinely necessary to protect their rights and well-being. If guardianship is denied, petitioners may consider appealing the decision or exploring alternative arrangements for support. Consulting with a legal professional experienced in guardianship matters may provide valuable guidance in addressing these issues.

PERSONAL EXPERIENCE WITH POWER OF ATTORNEY AND GUARDIANSHIP

In my 16 years as an administrator, power of attorney and guardianship has surfaced as a topic many times. Sometimes, the outcomes are difficult to navigate for the families involved as well as the healthcare personnel. For HIPPA compliance, I will not identify the names of people or facilities where these circumstances happened; however, I will share with you the events in which power of attorney and guardianship were very important.

On many occasions, as an administrator, during the natural aging process, some people lose their ability to swallow food naturally. The muscles in our bodies age, and sometimes, this affects the esophagus area. In skilled nursing, there is a speech therapy team. If the facility healthcare personnel observe difficulty in swallowing or pocketing food, a speech therapist will evaluate. They may order a swallow study. If it is recommended that the individual have a g-tube placed, the hospital healthcare personnel would then proceed with this surgery to place a g-tube for food to be given through a tube rather than swallowing. There are different types of tubes to feed individuals in this state. Healthcare personnel cannot decide to place a g-tube. Most of the time, individuals in this state cannot make their own decisions. At this time, healthcare personnel would rely on the family, surrogate, healthcare power of attorney or guardian to make this decision. This is a hefty decision. If one cannot eat, one cannot live.

There was a family at one of the locations where I was the administrator. Their loved one was recommended to have a g-tube placed by a speech therapist. The Power of attorney in place struggled greatly with this decision. Why, might you ask, was this a struggle? For this family, they were concerned the individual needing the g-tube would not be happy with this restriction, and his quality of life was at risk. Would **HE** want to live this way, being tube-fed for the rest of his life? Usually, this is not reversible, and people do not recover from this indicated method of feeding. I greatly respect this particular family because they were truly trying to make the decision he would make if he had the capacity to do so. Ultimately, they made the decision to place the feeding tube. As I would visit with this resident, there were very few times, I saw him smile. Did they make the right choice? I believe they did what they thought he would have wanted. These decisions are difficult and complex. Also, these decisions need to be made quickly. For the skilled nursing facility, we have to have a method of feeding an individual unless they are on hospice. This resident lived many years beyond this decision.

In another instance, a family member (power of attorney) chose not to have a feeding tube placed and then was immediately required to place his mother on hospice. As an administrator, I found this position very difficult. The nurses were outraged. They wanted to know how they could not feed this resident. Our whole motive in healthcare settings is to keep people alive. This ultimately would kill her. However, the part we are unaware of is what HER wishes would be if she could decide for herself. This was her son making the decision. Ultimately, he knows his mother better than anyone. Unfortunately, some of the healthcare personnel who were caring for this individual asked what were his motives? Was he going to gain anything financially? In this scenario, the son was the power of attorney for healthcare. He was given the power to make this decision by his mother – the patient. This story is included because I want you to know how powerful these decisions can be and how very closely they can affect the outcomes of what happens.

With this particular case, I consulted our legal and ethics team. Were we making the correct choices as healthcare professionals? The result was that the son had active healthcare power of attorney paperwork, and he ultimately had the final decision about the choice not to place a feeding tube. The mother passed away after about a month. Was she suffering? Our hospice team assured us that she was comfortable, but again, the nursing team continued to raise questions throughout this process. Our goal is always to keep people alive, but in this instance, we were required not to feed this individual who could not swallow on their own.

Unfortunately, in my line of work, when there is a death, and the person has money, property or something of value, it is often a family feud. It is so sad to see this. It is very often when there are assets. Very sadly, when there are no assets, there is very little fuss from families. I have seen both of these circumstances so many times. This book is not about a living will, but this can help in times when a loved one passes away so that it is clearly defined who will attain what assets. **Financial power of attorney ceases to be active at the time of a person's death.** There was a particular family at one location where the mother had five children. They were always visiting, which I greatly appreciated; however, an incident came up in which one of the daughters blamed my staff for taking an heirloom necklace. As an Administrator, this becomes an abuse investigation in which the person needs to be suspended pending investigation. I followed every policy and procedure as I always do. However, in the end, I believe it was the daughter who stated the necklace was missing and actually stole the heirloom necklace. She can be seen on video footage the night before this allegation, taking a large pile of clothing and other miscellaneous items out of the facility. Although this is very difficult to prove, every staff member must undergo a background check, for which there is no criminal history. Also, at the end of the investigation, who would want an heirloom necklace more than a family member? To make matters more complicated, the resident was confused and only spoke Italian. Some of these investigations get very complicated. As we are required to do, the local police were notified, but for something so small as this, they really rely on our information to help with their conclusion.

Other times when the power of attorney or guardianship comes into play are when the person is recommended for hospice or palliative care. This decision can be recommended by healthcare personnel, but ultimately, the power of attorney or surrogate decision-maker must make these decisions. Hospice and palliative care can offer a great number of additional support tools and comfort tools at the end of a person's life. Some Hospice companies provide pet therapy, music therapy, medications that are not otherwise allowed, and so much more. However, ultimately, this is the decision of the power of attorney or surrogate decision maker.

WHAT ARE ADVANCED DIRECTIVES?

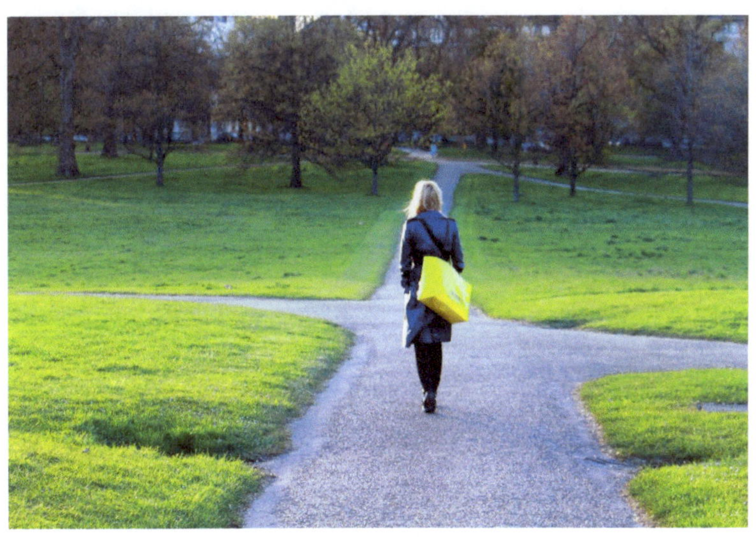

W hat about when a person is in an accident? What life-sustaining measures do they want in place? Do they want a ventilator? Do they want artificial measures to keep them alive? We are not talking about all advanced directives in this book, but it is important to know what they are.

What are Advanced Directives?

Advance directives are legal documents that allow individuals to express their preferences regarding medical treatment and healthcare decisions in the event that they become unable to communicate their wishes due to illness, injury, or incapacity. These documents are important for ensuring that a person's healthcare preferences are respected and followed by family members and medical providers. There are two primary types of advance directives:

1. Living Will:

A living will is a document that outlines an individual's preferences for medical treatment in situations where they are no longer able to make decisions for themselves, particularly regarding end-of-life care. Key aspects of a living will include:

- **Specific Treatments**: Directions on whether to accept or refuse specific medical treatments, such as resuscitation, mechanical ventilation, tube feeding, or other life-sustaining measures.
- **End-of-Life Wishes**: Guidelines for care preferences during terminal illness or irreversible conditions, focusing on comfort measures and palliative care.

2. Healthcare Power of Attorney (Healthcare Proxy):

This document designates a specific person (the agent or healthcare proxy) to make healthcare decisions on behalf of the individual if they become incapacitated. Key aspects of a healthcare power of attorney include:

- **Designation of Agent**: The individual chooses someone they trust to make medical decisions on their behalf, ensuring that decisions align with their values and preferences.
- **Authority**: The agent may have broad authority to make healthcare choices, including decisions about treatments, procedures, and end-of-life care.

Importance of Advance Directives:

- **Ensures Autonomy**: Advance directives allow individuals to maintain control over their medical treatment choices and ensure their wishes are respected, even if they are unable to communicate those wishes later.
- **Reduces Family Burden**: By clearly outlining preferences, advance directives can relieve family members from the emotional burden of making difficult decisions without guidance or consensus.
- **Guides Healthcare Providers**: Advance directives provide important information to healthcare professionals about a patient's preferences, allowing for more informed and respectful care.

Legal Considerations:

- **State-Specific Laws**: The requirements and validity of advance directives can vary by state, including how they must be executed, witnessed, or notarized. It's important to check state-specific laws when creating advance directives.
- **Regular Updates**: Individuals should regularly review and update their advance directives to ensure they reflect current wishes and circumstances, especially after significant life changes, such as marriage, divorce, or new medical diagnoses.

Conclusion:

Advance directives are vital components of healthcare planning that empower individuals to express their medical treatment preferences and designate decision-makers in the event of incapacity. Consulting with legal and healthcare professionals when creating advance directives can ensure that they are properly drafted and legally enforceable.

ADVANCED DIRECTIVES CAN INCLUDE A DNR OR (DO NOT RESUSCITATE) ORDER IF THE PERSON WISHES FOR THIS.

Is a DNR form part of advanced directives?

Yes, directives can include a Do Not Resuscitate (DNR) order, but they are typically considered separate documents that serve specific purposes within the broader context of advanced health-care planning.

Understanding DNR Orders:

1. **Do Not Resuscitate (DNR) Order:**
   - A DNR order is a medical order that instructs healthcare providers not to perform cardiopulmonary resuscitation (CPR) if a patient's heart stops beating or if they stop breathing.
   - DNR orders are often established for patients with terminal illnesses or severe health conditions where resuscitation would not be beneficial or in accordance with their wishes.

2. **Distinction from Advance Directives:**
   - While a DNR order can be part of a comprehensive advance directive, it is specifically focused on the decision to forego resuscitation efforts.
   - Advance directives, as mentioned earlier, include documents like living wills and healthcare powers of attorney, which outline broader healthcare preferences and designate decision-makers.

Incorporating a DNR into Advance Directives:

- Individuals may include their wishes regarding resuscitation in their advance directives, specifying whether they want a DNR order as part of their overall healthcare preferences.
- Depending on state laws, a separate DNR document may be required alongside other advance directives for the order to be recognized.

State-Specific Regulations:

- DNR orders are governed by state laws, and each state may have specific forms and procedures for establishing a DNR.
- It is crucial to understand the requirements in your state, including how to properly execute a DNR order and ensure it is honored by healthcare facilities.

Importance of Communication:

- Individuals should discuss their wishes regarding DNR orders and advance directives with family members, healthcare providers, and legal advisors to ensure clarity and understanding.

- Carrying a copy of the DNR order and advance directives in a readily accessible place can also facilitate honoring the individual's wishes during medical emergencies.

Conclusion:

While a DNR order is not the same as an advance directive, it can form an integral part of a person's overall healthcare plan. Individuals should ensure they understand their options, legal requirements, and healthcare preferences by consulting with healthcare and legal professionals when preparing these important documents.

CONCLUSION AND SUMMARY

Power of attorney and guardianship can be very useful documents when a person can no longer make their own decisions. There is a lot to consider among the choices that surround power of attorney and guardianship. As a healthcare personnel, I greatly urge families to have power of attorney in place before an individual can no longer make their own decisions. State guardians are very active in skilled nursing facilities when there is no one that can make decisions, and there is no surrogate decision maker. Power of attorney is not limited to a family member as the first choice. I once had a couple that had made their mailman their power of attorney. They had become close friends, and that was the individual they chose to handle their affairs when they could no longer make their own decisions. It just has to be decided ahead of time so that healthcare personnel know who is supposed to be making decisions, whether it be medical or financial.

About the Author

My name is Katie DeWerdt. I have three beautiful children and a fiancé. They keep me full of light and love on a daily basis. I enjoy reading, writing, exercising, doing outdoor activities, and spending time with family. I started writing books as a pastime in 2023. Besides this book, "Power of Attorney and Guardianship," you can also find my other books on Amazon, which are "Katie Cooks for You with Love" and "Getting Divorced Without Lawyers in the State of Illinois: a Beginner's Guide." If you type Katie DeWerdt in the Amazon search, all of my books will appear for purchase. Also, you can visit my website at https://katiecookswithlove.com to see all of my books for purchase.

For additional help with digital content, visit my web store at **https://sunshinedesign.store.**

You can also visit my YouTube channel **@KatieDeWerdt.**

To email me directly for any additional support or questions, please e-mail at **sunshinedesignstore@gmail.com**

www.ingramcontent.com/pod-product-compliance
Lightning Source LLC
Chambersburg PA
CBHW040851110726
48005CB00001B/18